# Dietary Chemicals vs. Dental Caries

Based on a Symposium on
Dietary Chemicals in Relation to
Dental Caries sponsored by
the Agricultural and Food Chemistry
Division at the 1966 Winter
Meeting of the American Chemical
Society, Phoenix, Arizona
January 18, 1966

**Robert S. Harris**
*Symposium Chairman*

ADVANCES IN CHEMISTRY SERIES **94**

AMERICAN CHEMICAL SOCIETY

WASHINGTON, D. C. 1970

Coden: ADCSHA



Library of Congress Catalog Card 71-142197

ISBN 8412-0108-0

PRINTED IN THE UNITED STATES OF AMERICA

# CONTENTS

Preface .......... vi

1. Dietary Chemicals in Relation to Dental Caries .......... 1
   Robert S. Harris

2. Carbohydrates, Fats, and Dental Caries .......... 7
   Ward Pigman

3. Amino Acids, Proteins, and Dental Caries .......... 23
   Abraham E. Nizel

4. Vitamins and Dental Caries .......... 33
   Samuel Dreizen

5. Antibiotics and Dental Caries .......... 46
   Basil G. Bibby

6. Other Organic Compounds and Dental Caries .......... 55
   Kenneth O. Madsen

7. Minerals: Fluorine and Dental Caries .......... 93
   Harold C. Hodge and Frank A. Smith

8. Minerals: Calcium and Phosphorus .......... 116
   Robert S. Harris

9. Effect of Minerals on Dental Caries .......... 123
   Juan M. Navia

10. Application of Chemical Agents for the Control of Dental Caries .. 161
    Robert C. Caldwell and Joe P. Thomas

Index .......... 181

# PREFACE

Dental Caries, a so-called "disease of civilization," seems to be worsening in the United States and appears to be related to the food that people eat. For these reasons, it seemed timely to hold a formal discussion of the factors that bear on the problem, and the symposium on "Dietary Chemicals in Relation to Dental Caries" was organized and presented at the Winter meeting of the American Chemical Society in 1966. Plans were laid from the beginning to publish this symposium, but absence of a critical paper on amino acids and proteins introduced delays. When Abraham E. Nizel, of the School of Dental Medicine, Tufts University, graciously accepted the invitation to fill this gap and submitted his paper in the Fall of 1968, the other authors were invited to up-date their papers. Subsequent review and revision has resulted in up-dating most of the papers to early or mid-1970. By the time his paper was ready for revision, Robert C. Caldwell had been appointed Dean of the School of Dentistry at the University of California, Los Angeles, and his colleague at the University of Alabama School of Dentistry, Joe P. Thomas, agreed to supervise the revision.

The resulting volume is a comprehensive and up-to-date survey of the major food-related factors that enter into tooth decay and its prevention. While it may not have all the answers, it does present the results on the major lines of effort on both cariogenic and cariostatic influences and will serve as a sound base for future research.

Robert S. Harris

Massachusetts Institute of Technology
Cambridge, Mass.
August 1970

1

# Dietary Chemicals in Relation to Dental Caries

ROBERT S. HARRIS

Massachusetts Institute of Technology, Cambridge, Mass.

*The incidence of dental caries and gingival and peridontal diseases is constantly increasing in the United States, although it varies with geographical location. Caries will not develop if the teeth are caries-resistant, if the mouth is kept clear of nutrients which support caries-producing bacteria, or if no caries-producing bacteria are present. Since permanent teeth begin to develop before two months of age, early nutrition may affect the eventual development of sound teeth. Various elements and compounds in food are classified as cariogenic or cariostatic. While caries in experimental animals is similar to that in man, caution is needed in projecting results of such studies.*

This symposium on "Dietary Chemicals in Relation to Dental Caries" was scheduled for presentation before the American Chemical Society because (a) the dental caries problem in the United States is serious, (b) many chemicals natural to foods have caries-producing or caries-preventing properties, (c) the caries activity of foods may be modified by processing or supplementation, (d) most of the literature relating to this subject has been published in journals which chemists (including food chemists) seldom peruse, and (e) it is important that chemists be informed of the potential importance of food chemicals in the control of dental decay.

More diseases afflict the mouth than any other part of the human body. Almost everyone in the United States is troubled with gingival and peridontal diseases and with dental caries at some time during his life span. In 1962, more than $2 billion was spent for dental services in the United States (9), a sum equivalent to about 1.5% of the national income and to about 15% of the total amount spent for health services (*14*). Though some 95,000 dentists are serving the U.S. population, less than 50% of the people have ever received dental care (*14*). At least twice as many dentists would be needed merely to correct current dental defects in the people.

The dental caries problem, which has been called a "disease of civilization," seems to be worsening. For instance, Bartholdi *et al.* (*1*) noted that the number of caries-free subjects among entering freshmen at the University of Minnesota decreased from 1.8 to 1.3% between 1929 and 1959, and the incidence of carious teeth rose from 34.8 to 49.3%. It is likely that similar trends are developing relative to disorders of the soft tissues of the mouth. Kite and Swanson (*6*) recently reported the results of a survey of the modern dental care provided to freshmen at the Massachusetts Institute of Technology. One in four among the 913 students between 16 and 20 years old examined had incipient gingival disease, and the average DMFT (decayed, missing, and filled teeth) rate was 9.6. Detectable tooth decay was being controlled in only 42% of the students, and few of these had received needed periodontal care. Orthodontic care was received by only 18% of the students, and this was during an average of 2.9 years. Depending upon the criteria used, malocclusion occurred in 61 to 71% of those students who still had all permanent teeth.

The geography of dental caries in the United States (Figure 1) is interesting (*2*). It is highest in the Northeast, next highest in the North-

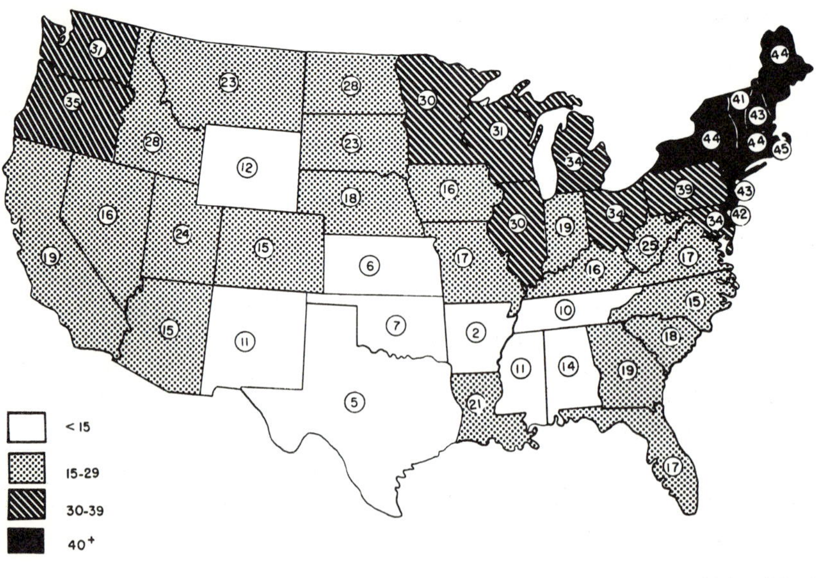


J. M. Dunning, "Dental Clinics of North America," Saunders

*Figure 1. Incidence and distribution of dental caries*

west and North-Central area, and least in the South-Central area. The higher incidence of caries in the areas of higher rainfall has led some to suggest that the leaching of minerals from the soil may be a controlling factor in caries development in this country. While it is true that rain water will slowly remove minerals from the soil and consequently reduce the mineral content of local water supplies and of food plants grown on these soils, the interesting geography of caries in the United States cannot be explained this simply.

Foods and nutrition have important effects upon oral health. The observation that dental caries does not develop in germ-free animals fed sterilized diets (*11*) indicates that bacteria are essential to the tooth decay process. The demonstration that caries does not develop in normal animals fed by gastric intubation (*5*) indicates that residues of food debris are needed in the mouth to supply nutrients for the growth and development of caries-producing bacteria.

It is pointed out in this symposium that many elements and compounds in foods may accelerate or reduce the development of dental caries (*8*). Dietary deficiencies of vitamins (*e.g.*, A, $B_6$, $B_{12}$, D, E, riboflavin, niacin), minerals (*e.g.*, Ca, P, Fe, Mn), and amino acids (*e.g.*, lysine, tryptophan) interfere with the development and maintenance of healthy tissues in the mouth. Because oral tissues are sensitive and convenient for observation, nutritional clinicians routinely examine the mouth when appraising the nutrition status of human beings.

Some minerals are cariogenic, some are cariostatic, and some are inert when ingested in the diet. The bran layers of cereals contain organic compounds that have cariostatic properties, yet on occasion this "roughage" may act as a local irritant to the gingiva. Sucrose is cariogenic, glucose is relatively inert, and starch is inert. Many other elements and compounds may be cited to demonstrate that the presence and absence of nutrients and nonnutrients in foods play a major role in determining the health of oral tissues.

Nutrients and other chemicals in foods may affect the teeth through three routes: by reacting with the tooth surface as the food passes through the mouth (local action), by reacting with the tooth surface after being absorbed from the intestine and returned to the mouth *via* the saliva and then reacting with the tooth surface (systemic-local action), and after being absorbed from the intestine and entering the tooth in the circulating blood (systemic action).

The systemic influences of nutritional factors upon the teeth are greatest during tooth development. The periodontium is continually under the influence of systemic factors from the time of eruption of the first tooth until the death of the host. The growth, development, and maintenance of oral tissues are influenced by nutrition because cell growth and metabolism, protein synthesis, and calcification processes are involved. Disturbances in protein metabolism may influence matrix formation in the enamel and dentin of the developing tooth, as well as the intercellular matrix of the cementum, the fibrous periodontal membrane, and the alveolar bone. Faults in the metabolism of carbohydrates and fats may alter vital reactions in the cells of these tissues. Deficiencies of vitamin A may affect the formation of enamel matrix and the maintenance of the epithelium of the periodontal tissue; vitamin C deficiency may affect the formation of the collagen matrix in dentin, cementum, periodontal membrane, and alveolar bone; vitamin D deficiency may affect the calcification of enamel, dentin, cementum, and alveolar bone, etc. Deficiencies and excesses of minerals may affect the composition of the calcified tissues, or may alter cell metabolism through their role in co-enzymes (*3*).

These systemic influences are joined by local effects when the tooth erupts into the oral cavity. Ion exchange reactions with the surfaces of the oral tissues by elements and compounds present in the saliva and pulp fluids become important. Degradation products of dietary carbohydrates and microbial enzymes on the surfaces of the tooth can promote caries development. Recent research has demonstrated that certain types of mucopolysaccharide-producing microorganisms which require sucrose for their metabolism may be the major cause of dental caries in human beings.

At least three factors (Figure 2) are involved in the development of dental caries: host and teeth, microflora, and substrate in the mouth (*4*). Caries will not develop if the teeth are caries-resistant, if the mouth is kept cleared of nutrients (especially sucrose) which will sustain the growth and metabolism of caries-producing bacteria, or if the mouth is not infected with caries-producing bacteria. Thus, caries can be controlled by altering only one of these conditions.

The age of the tooth is important. Caries in deciduous teeth may cause early tooth loss and affect the positioning of the permanent teeth which are developing below. Dental caries in the permanent dentition is of major importance because these teeth are "permanent" and are irretrievable if lost through neglect. Though deciduous teeth are generally lost by 11 years of age, the permanent teeth begin to develop before 2 months of age. Thus, nutrition may have an effect upon the growth and development of a sound tooth long before it has erupted into the mouth.

The earliest visible sign of caries is characterized by porous, chalky white spots in the enamel. The "smooth surface" type of caries shows a wide-angled wedge of penetration. The "pit-and-fissure" caries develop a wedge of decay that is sharper and inverted, with the point at the surface.

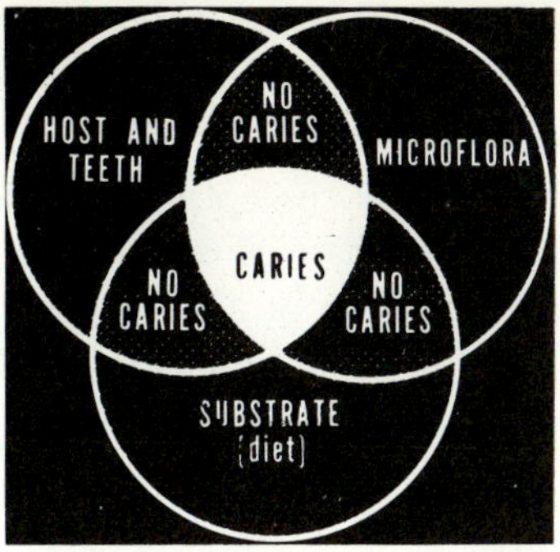


P. H. Keyes and H. V. Jordan, "Mechanisms of Hard Tissue Destruction," American Association for the Advancement of Science

*Figure 2. Factors responsible for caries activity*

In either case, the shape of the lesion corresponds with the direction of the enamel rods, indicating that the path of penetration of decay follows structural pathways. Once the surface of the enamel has been destroyed, the bacterial invasion proceeds along an uneven front following the enamel rod pattern.

Dentinal caries develops as a disorganization of the matrix, and in the direction of incremental growth lines, causing first a lateral spread, and later a progression along the dentinal tubules.

The rat has been used most widely in experimental caries research. The deep fissures in the molar teeth show the highest incidence and extent of dental caries development. While these carious lesions are very similar to those in man, no experimental animal has teeth that completely resemble those of the human being. Thus, the results of caries research conducted with rats, hamsters, and even primates cannot be projected to the human being without reservation.

During the development of caries, minerals may be withdrawn from considerable depths in the tooth structure, in spite of the high density of the enamel (*12*). Demineralizing agents reach into the enamel structure along pathways related primarily to the striated structure of the enamel.

Dental caries has been reported to develop in experimental animals within four days following eruption (*13*). Opdyke (*10*) has studied the time-sequence of lesions produced artificially in human tooth enamel that is being exposed to an acidic salivary–glucose–agar system *in vitro*. The first reaction was a release of free mineral after four days' exposure; within eight days the lesion had a characteristic acid reaction (pH 4.2–4.5); after the 10th day various amino acid fractions were observed, and, finally, after 20 days lipid substances were found.

Since the structure of the tooth is important to the pathogenesis of caries, those factors which influence the structure of teeth during development are especially important. Mellanby (7) has been foremost in promoting the concept that the high susceptibility to caries in modern man results from the faulty tooth structure caused by diet abnormalities during tooth development.

Finally, it should be emphasized that caries development is catalyzed or retarded by the presence of elements and compounds, both nutrients and nonnutrients, which act systemically or locally. These are the subject of this symposium.

*Acknowledgment*

Contribution Number 1429 from the Department of Nutrition and Food Science, Massachusetts Institute of Technology, Cambridge, Mass.

*Literature Cited*

(1) Bartholdi, W. L., Peterson, E. E., Crawford, W. H., *J. Am. Dental Assoc.* **1961,** 63, 868–871.
(2) Dunning, J. M., "The Dental Clinics of North America," pp. 291–303, Saunders, Philadelphia, Pa., 1962.
(3) Harris, R. S., Ed., "The Art and Science of Dental Caries Research," Academic, New York, 1968.
(4) Keyes, P. H., Jordan, H. V., "Mechanisms of Hard Tissue Destruction," R. F. Sognnaes, Ed., pp. 261–283, Pub. 75, American Association for the Advancement of Science, Washington, D. C., 1963.
(5) Kite, O. W., Shaw, J. H., Sognnaes, R. F., *J. Nutr.* **1950,** 42, 89–103.
(6) Kite, Owen W., Swanson, Leonard T., *J. Am. Dental Assoc.* **1965,** 70, 1143–1152.
(7) Mellanby, M., "The effect of diet on dental structure and disease in man," Medical Research Council, Spec. Rept. Ser. #191, London, 1936.
(8) Nizel, A. E., "The Science of Nutrition and Its Application in Clinical Dentistry," A. E. Nizel, Ed., Saunders, Philadelphia, Pa., 1966.
(9) Office of Business Economics, "Survey of Current Business," U. S. Dept. of Commerce, Washington, D. C., July 1963.
(10) Opdyke, D. L., *J. Dental Res.* **1960,** 39, 698, Abst. 129.
(11) Orland, F. J., Blayney, J. R., Harrison, R. W., Reyniers, J. A., Trexler, P. C., Gordon, H. A., Wagner, M., Luckey, T. D., *J. Dental Res.* **1954,** 33, 147–174.
(12) Sognnaes, R. F., "Chemistry and Prevention of Dental Caries," Charles C. Thomas, Springfield, Ill., 1962.
(13) Steinman, R. R., Hewes, C. G., Woods, R. W., *J. Dental Res.* **1959,** 38, 592–605.
(14) Volker, J. F., "Dental Clinics of North America," p. 385, Saunders, Philadelphia, Pa., 1962.

RECEIVED October 27, 1969.

# 2

# Carbohydrates, Fats, and Dental Caries

WARD PIGMAN

Department of Biochemistry, New York Medical College,
New York, N. Y. 10029

*Dental caries results from attack on the tooth surface by microorganisms, especially in noncleansing areas. Dietary factors may influence this attack by acting on the tooth or the microorganisms. With experimental animals, dietary carbohydrates exert a pre- and post-eruptive cariogenic effect, whereas fats as a whole may mediate the post-eruptive effect. Comparisons of primitive man with man living under urban conditions have demonstrated a great enhancement in dental caries in modern man. Such studies and those with controlled populations have suggested that some types of carbohydrates are the main origin of the increased incidence of dental decay.* In vitro *studies using the artificial mouth have shown most common sugars to be potentially cariogenic.*

Carbohydrate constituents usually provide the major source of energy in human diets. As starches, modified starches, and sugars, they also have been the dietary products most susceptible to industrial modification and application in products such as syrups, refined sugars, candies, gums, puddings, soft drinks, canned fruits, and other products. Since these products are produced and consumed mainly in highly industrialized countries, which also have high rates of dental decay, much interest has been shown in the relationship of such products to dental caries. Many investigations of various types have been carried out to determine whether a direct relationship exists between dietary carbohydrates and the incidence of dental caries. The number of such investigations is so great that they cannot be considered adequately in this review. As a result, the principal types of investigations will be considered, and except for recent work, reference generally will be given to secondary sources which discuss the subject more adequately and also give the original literature. A valuable bibliography of recent research on dental caries has been prepared by Brislin and Cox (*4*).

Universal agreement seems to exist on the nature of the basic process involved in dental caries. It consists of the attack by the products of metabolism of oral bacteria on exposed surfaces of teeth, usually on enamel, but also occurring on cementum and exposed dentin. The attack is thus basically external, although possibly modified by internal metabolic influences. Dental caries initially is nearly always highly localized and in positions which are noncleansing. The distribution of lesions in the mouth has a similar pattern in most persons, and the areas most commonly affected are the pits and fissures of molars and premolars, interproximal positions, and cervical margins. These positions accumulate food particles, and presumably are the best positions for the establishment of bacterial plaques. The combination of food material and bacteria provide the attack factor in dental caries. The attack, however, is modified by many factors, some of which will be considered later.

Saliva is related to dental caries as a biological fluid which washes out fermentable substrates before they are metabolized, dilutes harmful bacterial products before they attack the tooth surface, possibly repairs incipient carious lesions through remineralization, and modifies the tooth surface by providing the elements needed for the secondary cuticle of the tooth. In addition, its immune bodies may affect the bacterial population.

### *Pre-Eruptive and Systemic Effects*

Relatively little is known, except concerning fluorides, of the dietary effects that take place during tooth formation or which result from general metabolic influences. However, Kite, Shaw, and Sognnaes (*23, 30*) showed that rats fed on carbohydrate-rich diets developed caries, but a group to which the same diet was given by stomach tube developed no caries. This indicates that the effect was primarily a local one at the tooth surface.

Several studies have been carried out with different types of animals given high-carbohydrate diets at various stages of tooth formation and maturation (*23, 28*). Sognnaes (Table I) found that animals fed such diets during pregnancy had progeny with higher caries susceptibility than those fed "natural" diets. Since the individual molar teeth of rats and hamsters are formed and erupt at different periods, the effect of a high-carbohydrate diet during the period of tooth formation and subsequent maturation also could be studied. These experiments showed the existence of a period of high caries susceptibility following eruption of the teeth and a gradual maturation to a less susceptible condition [Finn, Klapper and Volker (*28*)].

**Table I. Comparison of Caries Susceptibility in Hamsters, Rats, and Mice When "Bred" on Stock Diet *vs.* Purified Diet**[a]

| *Species* | *No. of Animals* | *Pregnancy and Lactation* | *Posteruptive Diet* | *Posteruptive Period, Months* | *Average Caries Incidence Molars Affected* | *Average Caries Incidence Areas Affected* | *Average Caries Incidence Caries Score* |
|---|---|---|---|---|---|---|---|
| Hamsters | 6 | Stock | Purified | 4 | 4.6 | 5.3 | 6.1 |
| Rats | 12 | Stock | Purified | 4 | 0 | 0 | 0 |
| Mice | 15 | Stock | Purified | 4 | 0 | 0 | 0 |
| Hamsters | 3 | Purified | Purified | 2 | 9.0 | 31.6 | 48.0 |
| Rats | 10 | Purified | Purified | 2 | 2.4 | 2.7 | 2.7 |
| Mice | 21 | Purified | Purified | 2 | 0.4 | 0.5 | 0.5 |

[a] From Sognnaes (*30*). Copyright by the American Dental Association. Reprinted by permission.

The effects of prenatal nutrition on the oral structures have been reviewed by Larson (*19*). Shaw and Griffiths (*26, 27*) reported many malformed third molars in young rats whose mothers had been on diets with a protein-to-sucrose ratio of 8:83, as compared with those from mothers having a ratio of 24:67. Halloway *et al.* (*15*), in addition to morphological changes, found that the young of mother rats on a high-sucrose diet had teeth less resistant to caries.

### *Effects on Mature Teeth*

Three general procedures have been used for studies of the influence of dietary carbohydrates and fats on the incidence of tooth decay. These are human nutritional studies with groups having different diets, animal studies with controlled diets, and *in vitro* procedures. These will be discussed separately.

**Human Nutritional Studies** (*1, 23, 30*). Many studies have been made using human populations. These include institutionalized people on controlled diets, persons on restricted diets (diabetics, for example), and people living under conditions not affected by modern industrialization (*e.g.*, Eskimos, Indians, etc.). Such studies are difficult to conduct and to interpret in relation to causal relationships. They show that generally persons living under primitive conditions have low caries rates; the same population types living in urban areas with contact with modern industrial products have much higher average rates of caries. Since many factors are different for such urban and rural conditions, a direct relation to dietary constituents cannot be demonstrated.

One human study requires special attention. This study was carried out at the Vipeholm Mental Hospital at Lund, Sweden, and has become known as the Vipeholm Dental Caries Study (*20, 32*). This carefully conducted study showed a fairly clear relationship between carbohydrate products of some types and dental caries experience. It will be discussed in more detail in a later section.

The effects of fats in human dietary studies have been summarized by Volker and Caldwell (*35*). The general impression is that diets rich in fats are low in cariogenicity. Thus, nomadic Eskimos on protein–fat diets, composed of as much as 65% fat, had low caries incidence. The results of several clinical studies on controlled groups were interpreted similarly, but, as with most of the studies on high-carbohydrate diets, the interpretations have questionable significance.

**Animal Studies** (*28*). Many studies of dietary composition in relation to dental caries have been carried out with experimental animals. Hamsters and rats have been used principally, but monkeys and other animals also have been employed. The carious lesions produced in rats and hamsters seem to be similar to those produced in humans, although in the early work with rats the caries seemed to be related to coarse diets and the formation of cracks in the tooth structure. The caries rate can be greatly increased by prior removal of the main salivary glands.

The use of "natural diets" such as Purina Chow usually resulted in low caries rates. When a major part of the diet was composed of starches, sucrose, or dextrose, dental caries was extensive, although some studies have found starches and dextrins to be less cariogenic than sucrose or dextrose [*See* Finn, Klapper, and Volker (*28*)]. Klapper and Volker found fructose and especially sorbitol to be less cariogenic than sucrose. McClure (*28*) found that the cariogenic effect of milk products and processed cereals could be greatly increased by heat treatments. These results, arising from destruction of lysine, emphasize the need for knowledge of the effects of processing treatments on the possible cariogenicity of food products. The cariogenicity of dry whey powders also suggests that lactose is probably cariogenic in animal experiments.

Instead of experimental diets, Stephan (*31*) added human foods (53 in all) to basic diets of rats and compared the caries experience to that of animals receiving diets of known cariogenicity. As a result, he classified food products into five groups, according to the amount of caries. The most extreme group was composed of foods rich in carbohydrates, especially fermentable sugars.

The interpretation of animal experiments of this type in terms of human caries is fraught with difficulties. The caries rate is very high as compared with the usual human rate. One factor increasing the rate is the small size of rodent teeth and the resulting thin enamel. Another is the constant "dirty" mouth; such animals usually have the teeth buried in solid food particles. This factor is even more drastic in desalivated animals, which also introduces the problem of comparisons of starches with sucrose or dextrose in the absence of salivary amylases. The animal diets usually include starch as uncooked particles, different from the gelatinized starches common for human diets. For animal experiments of this type, the attack forces could overwhelm any mild protective forces such as possible saliva components or anatomical relations. Thus, Haldi *et al.* (*13*) found that in hamsters a high sucrose diet produced a larger caries score than a similar diet with glucose, but for desalivated animals, the two diets gave similar results.

Another major difficulty is that the various laboratories pass through periods during which the usual cariogenic diets do not produce the expected caries. This variability is probably explained by the observation of Fitzgerald and Keyes [McDonald (*28*)] that caries-inactive rodents could be converted to caries-active animals by exposure to caries-active animals or their feces. Thus, an appropriate oral flora is required for caries production. Earlier, Orland had demonstrated that germ-free rats did not acquire caries when fed diets normally cariogenic.

Several studies of the effects of dietary fats on caries incidence in rats or hamsters have been summarized by Volker (*34*). The fats included were corn oil, lard, arachis oil, and hydrogenated arachis oil. These studies showed a reduced incidence of caries in comparison with the control diets. Since the fats reduced the other components of the diet, the effect may not have been cariostatic, but instead the result of dilution of a cariogenic component. The usual interpretation of these experiments has been that the fats favored oral clearance, perhaps by forming films on the teeth.

### In Vitro *Laboratory Procedures*

A number of laboratory procedures have been used to investigate the possible cariogenicity of carbohydrates and foodstuffs.

**Acid Production and Plaque pH** (*35*). When human salivas, salivary debris, or salivary microorganisms are incubated with many sugars, starch products, or foodstuffs containing these carbohydrates, the solutions rapidly become acidic (usually pH 4.5–5.0). Starch products appear to produce acid more slowly than the common sugars.

A modification of this method for *in vivo* studies was described by Stephan. Human subjects were instructed not to brush their teeth for several days. The pH of tooth surfaces was then measured by touching the teeth with a tiny electrode (antimony or glass) and with a calomel electrode contacting the saliva in the floor of the mouth. The mouth then was rinsed with a solution containing a carbohydrate or suspended foodstuff. The pH of the plaque was measured at short time intervals. With the common sugars, a rapid decrease of pH occurred, followed usually by a slow return to the original pH. Results given by Ludwig and Bibby (*29*) are shown in Figure 1.

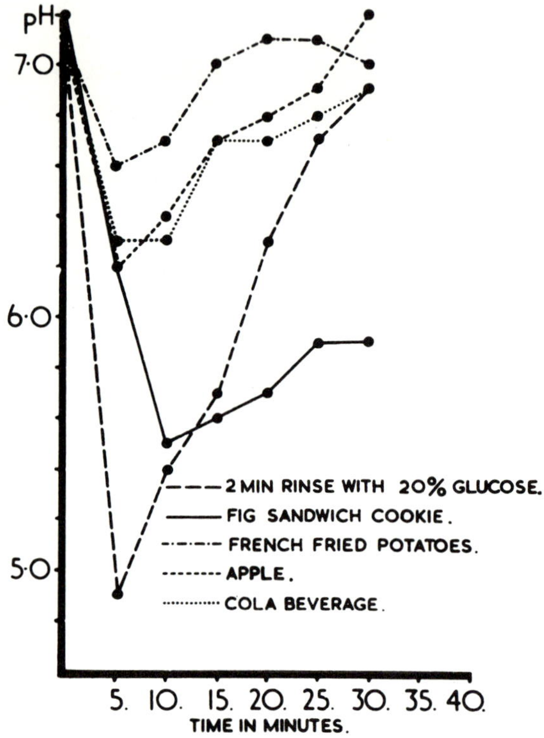


From Sognnaes, R. F., Ed., "Chemistry and Prevention of Dental Caries," 1962. Courtesy of Charles C. Thomas, Publisher, Springfield, Illinois.

*Figure 1. Effect of various foods on plaque pH, based on data by Ludwig and Bibby; taken from Jenkins* (29)

The actual results have varied somewhat in various investigations using different conditions. The general pattern is for sugars such as dextrose and sucrose to show a rapid pH drop of several units and rapid recovery. Starch products and foods may show a less marked decrease and often a slower recovery.

Recent studies of plaque pH changes by G. Frostel (*2*) after ingestion of sorbitol and hydrogenated dextrin products indicate that these products induced less pH change than sucrose. However, Caldwell and

Bibby (*6*) showed that the pH of carious lesions (rather than plaque pH) increased when some foodstuffs were taken by mouth.

The significance of these results in terms of the relation of human diets to human caries experience is uncertain. If the assumption is made that the production of organic acids by oral bacteria is an important feature of the carious process, the results do provide a means for demonstration of the possible cariogenic effects of dietary components. However, as carried out, the results are at best only semiquantitative and capable of demonstration of only gross differences. They do suggest, however, the inadvisability of maintaining continuously high levels of fermentable carbohydrates in the saliva.

***In Vitro* Caries Production** (*24*). The enamel covering the crown of human teeth is without cells and is incapable of restoration except by purely chemical exchange with salivary components. The caries process in enamel may be reproducible by purely *in vitro* procedures except for secondary effects, such as deposition of secondary dentin (*24*). The many earlier *in vitro* experiments begun by Magitot (1870) and other workers terminated in the development of the artificial mouth (*24*).

The operation of the artificial mouth consists basically of exposure of mounted extracted human teeth to saliva and subsequently to a bacteriological medium which maintains the metabolism of the oral microorganisms on the tooth surface. The teeth may be brushed regularly to simulate natural lesions, and pure strains of microorganisms may be used. For quantitative comparisons, blocks of human enamel may be used instead of whole teeth and the softening which results from the caries

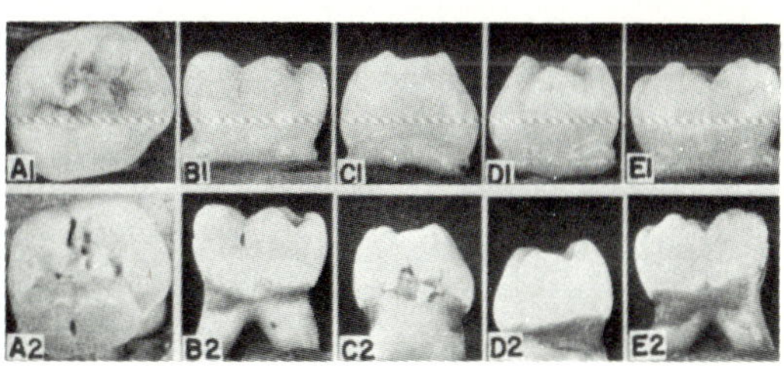


Journal of the American Dental Association

*Figure 2. Pattern of carious attack on lower left second deciduous molar* (24)

*A1, Occlusal aspect; B1, buccal aspect; C1, mesial aspect; D1, distal aspect; and E1, lingual aspect before the tooth was put on the standard regime. A2, B2, C2, D2, and E2 show the respective surfaces after 9 weeks on the standard regime.*

production can be followed by microhardness measurements. Typical lesions produced in a brushed molar are shown in Figure 2.

The following carbohydrates were tested for their ability to cause the softening of enamel surfaces in the presence of oral microorganisms: dextrose, fructose, galactose, lactose, maltose, sucrose, and soluble starch. The soluble starch caused no softening, but the sugars, with the possible exception of maltose, showed comparable rates of softening (*25*). 3-*O*-methyl-D-fructose and 3-*O*-methyl-D-glucose were not fermented by oral microorganisms, but 3-*O*-methyl-D-glucose was a neurotoxic agent.

An interesting relation between sugar concentration and the type of attack was observed when the concentration of D-glucose (dextrose) in the bacteriological medium was studied (*24*). With sugar added to the bacteriological medium, decalcified dentin was attacked but not sound enamel or dentin; the attack was thus proteolytic in nature. With 0.5% dextrose in the medium, sound enamel and dentin were extensively decalcified, but no attack on decalcified dentin was observed. For 0.2 to 0.3% solutions, dentinal matrix was attacked and decalcification of sound enamel and dentin occurred. These results suggest in terms of human oral conditions that the concentration of fermentable sugar in the saliva will determine the nature of the carious attack, which may vary at different times during the day.

The artificial mouth has been used for tests of the cariogenicity of foodstuffs. Koulourides (unpublished data) suspended breakfast cereals (corn base) in water and used this as the bacteriological medium.

The principal question with regard to this procedure is whether the microbial population is truly representative of the real flora of the oral cavity. The attack rate is considerably faster than that usually observed in the human mouth.

### *Oral Clearance Studies and Food Retention*

Clinical dentists generally have associated caries lesions with noncleansing areas of teeth and the resulting accumulation of food particles. Such areas also would tend to favor formation of bacterial plaques. In recent years, many laboratory investigations into the factors affecting the rate of removal of food products from the mouth have been carried out. These have been reviewed by Volker and Caldwell (*35*). The principal studies have been carried out by direct measurements of the amount of food residues after various times of chewing, by measurements of the amount of salivary reducing sugar during and after digestion of food, and by measurements of properties of foods (such as adhesion) which would be expected to affect food retention.

Bibby and associates (*35*) have studied the retention of food particles in the mouth during chewing and have compared various food products. They also measured the acid formed by the foods when incubated with saliva, and established a "Decalcification Potential" based on both measurements. Fig cookies, dates, chocolates, and ice cream were retained in highest amounts, and potato chips and carrots (cooked and uncooked) were cleared the most rapidly of the foods studied.

Caldwell (*5, 35*) developed an apparatus to measure the adhesion of food products to tooth enamel *in vitro.* The results for a wide range of foods showed that the foods had markedly different adhesive properties. Caramels and toffe (a hard candy) were the most adhesive foods.

Volker and Pinkerton (1947) first used salivary reducing sugar as a measure of food retention by human subjects (*33*). It was used also by Lundqvist (*20*) as part of the comprehensive Vipeholm study (*32*) and later by Lanke (*18*) in an extension of the Vipeholm study to oral clearance studies of foods. Table II from Volker (*33*), shows the salivary reducing sugar levels after ingestion of several foodstuffs.

**Table II. Reducing Sugar (as D-Glucose) in Human Saliva[a] after Ingestion of Several Foods or Confections[b]**

| *Substance* | *No. of Subjects* | *Time of Eating, Min.* | *Av. Glucose Conc. in mg. %* 0 *Time*[c] | 5 *Min.*[d] | 15 *Min.*[d] | 30 *Min.*[d] |
|---|---|---|---|---|---|---|
| Chewing gum, Dentyne, 3.2 grams | 28 | 30 (chewing) | 19 | 484 | 147 | 26 |
| Soft mint, Birch Bit, 2.5 grams | 12 | 4 | 16 | 662 | 131 | 23 |
| Hard mint, Toronto Mint, 1.9 grams | 12 | 9 (av.) | 21 | 377 | 259 | 24 |
| Chewy candy, Chocletto, 5.9 grams | 11 | 7 | 24 | 1,909 | 269 | 26 |
| Cookie, vanilla wafer, 8.2 grams | 12 | 2.5 | 16 | 889 | 117 | 18 |
| Bread and jam, 76.0 grams | 12 | 3 | 25 | 1,475 | 149 | 22 |

[a] Reducing substances in saliva calculated as glucose.

[b] From Volker (*33*). Copyright by the American Dental Association. Reprinted by permission.

[c] Zero time value is control value taken immediately before beginning the ingestion of the test substances.

[d] Time intervening since the beginning of ingestion of the test substances.

### *The Vipeholm Dental Caries Study*

The Vipeholm Dental Caries Study was certainly the best designed and conducted and the freest of criticism of all clinical studies of the direct effect of foodstuffs on caries incidence in humans. Institutionalized mental patients (436) under close supervision and control were used principally. Two studies, each of 2 years' duration, followed 2 years of preparation and preliminary studies. Seven groups were formed, all with a basic diet plus supplements:

(1) Control Group on basic diet with 150 grams or 40 grams of margarine as caloric compensation for carbohydrates added in other diets.

(2) Sucrose Group given sucrose in solution at meals.

(3) Bread Group given sugar-rich bread or rolls.

(4) Chocolate Group given sucrose in solution for first 2 years and milk chocolate for the last 2 years.

(5) Caramel Group given sugar-rich bread the first year, caramels the next 2 years, and no supplement the last year.

(6) 8-Toffee Group given no supplement the first year and 8 toffees (hard candies) daily for 3 years.

(7) 24-Toffee Group given 24 toffees daily for 1.5 years and no supplement for the last 2.5 years.

The basic diet for the first 2 years was 1800 calories, low in sugars but having considerable bread and potatoes as carbohydrate sources. The basic diet for the last 2 years provided 2700 calories, and the amounts of bread and potatoes were increased particularly. The vitamin and mineral content were studied and considered satisfactory. Candies, when given in addition to the basic diet, apparently could be eaten between meals. The carbohydrate consumption by groups was recorded. Careful dental examinations were carried out annually, with two examinations prior to the study.

Some of the results are as follows. When the sugar was consumed only at meals and the total amount consumed was compared with dental caries experiences, practically no relation could be demonstrated, and the caries rate was low. When the candies were given between meals, a marked enhancement of rate was demonstrated over the control group. When the candies were removed, the rates dropped again in the subsequent period.

The conclusions of the study are:

(1) The consumption of sugar can increase caries activity.

(2) The risk of sugar increasing caries activity is great if the sugar is consumed in a form with a strong tendency to be retained on the surface of the teeth.

(3) The risk of sugar increasing caries activity is greatest if the sugar is consumed between meals and in a form in which the tendency to be

retained on the surface of the teeth is pronounced, with a transiently high concentration of sugar on these surfaces.

(4) The increase in caries activity under uniform experimental conditions varies widely from one person to another.

(5) Increase in caries activity due to intake of sugar-rich foodstuffs consumed in a manner favoring caries disappears on withdrawal of such foodstuffs from the diet.

(6) Caries lesions may continue to appear despite the avoidance of refined sugar and maximum restriction of natural sugars and total dietary carbohydrates.

By sugar, sucrose was meant, and the study seemed to evaluate primarily the effects of candies taken between meals. Sugars taken normally at meals had little influence. Starch products were not considered.

The significance of the study was considerably enhanced by a parallel study by Lundqvist (*20*) of the same groups. For this study, the salivary reducing sugars (after acid hydrolysis of saliva samples) were measured at 15-minute periods during the working hours on typical days for the seven groups. These studies showed increases between meals, and with some persons the salivas almost continuously had glucose equivalents of 0.3 to 2%. The salivary reducing sugar profiles for the various groups are shown in Figure 3. The figure also gives the caries activity of the groups.

The individual patterns of salivary reducing sugar were quantitated by calculation of a clearance time based on the reducing sugar concentration and percentage of the waking hours involved. These clearance times for the various groups correlated closely with the caries activity, as shown in Figure 4.

In a separate study using two persons, Lundqvist (*20, 35*) also measured the clearance of a large number of foods by measuring the salivary reducing sugar (after acid hydrolysis) over a period of time. The results did not correlate always with the total carbohydrate content, although candies and sugar-rich products were given the highest caries potentiality index.

Although the physical consistency of foods generally has been related to carbohydrate oral clearance, recent work has indicated that the elimination of solid foods from diets of rodents resulted in a rapid decrease of salivary gland function and gland weight (*14*). In addition to food clearance and salivary gland atrophy, a third factor has been suggested as contributing to higher tooth resistance against caries. This is the mechanical effect of mastication on the crystallites of the enamel structure (*21*). Although direct evidence for this factor is lacking, it may be an additional mechanism relating the physical consistency of foods to the development of dental caries.

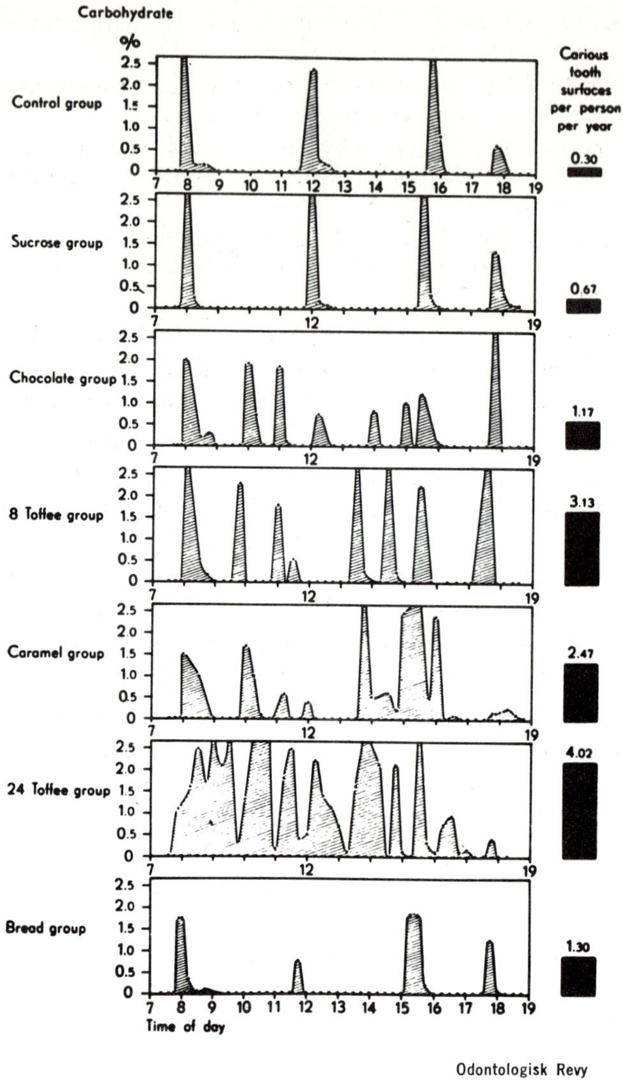


*Figure 3. Concentrations of salivary reducing sugar during the waking periods of persons in the seven groups of the Vipeholm Study as given by Lundqvist* (20)

### *The Place of Sucrose*

Sucrose is one of the most important industrial sugars used in foods. Although most of the early studies cited previously did not differentiate sucrose from other commercial sugars and starches, considerable recent work suggests that it may be more cariogenic. This recent work has been reviewed by Newbrun (*22*). The basis for the special effect is the relationship of the cariogenicity of streptococci and some other microorganisms to their ability to form bacterial plaques and extracellular dextrans and levans. Experimentally, these polysaccharides are formed from sucrose but not from glucose or other common sugars. These polysaccharides apparently aid plaque growth by helping the microorganisms to attach themselves to the enamel surface. They may act also as a storage form of fructose or glucose which may be released slowly between meals.

Gustafson *et al.* (*12*) early showed that the caries activity of experimental diets for hamsters was related to the sucrose content. Krasse (*17*) found that sucrose was better than glucose in inducing plaques of caries-inducing streptococci. The inclusion of sucrose in animal diets caused the production of both extracellular and intracellular polysaccharides, whereas glucose caused the formation of only intracellular material (*9*).

Rats or hamsters which had their indigenous oral flora depressed by the use of antibiotics were inoculated with cariogenic streptococci. Diets containing 25% of the following carbohydrates were used: sucrose, glucose, fructose, maltose, and uncooked starch. The streptococci did not survive in animals fed on diets lacking in sucrose, and the highest caries experience was found for the group given sucrose (*8, 11*).

In other similar studies, but with natural oral flora, on rats fed diets in which a number of carbohydrates were compared with sucrose, the results were more equivocal. All of the sugars produced comparable caries, at least in some experiments (*10, 26, 27*).

With monkeys on carbohydrate-restricted diets, Bowen and Cornick (*3*) found that the oral population of bacteria which formed polysaccharides decreased and increased when carbohydrates were incorporated into the diets.

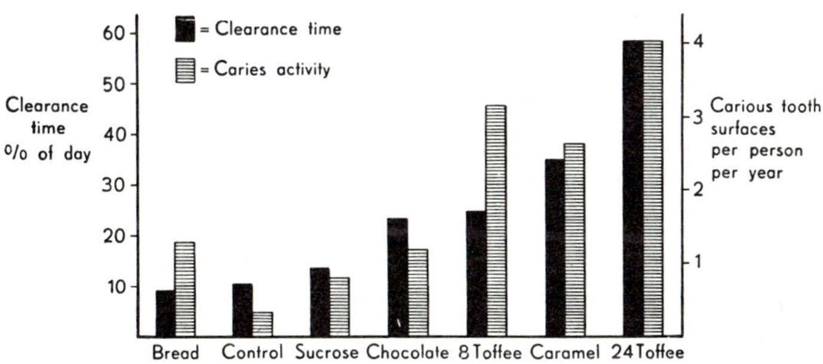


Odontologisk Revy

*Figure 4. Comparison of clearance of reducing sugar from the saliva of persons in the Vipeholm Study (Lundqvist, 20)*

### *Present Status*

**Basis of Variability of Caries Experience.** One of the conclusions of the Vipeholm study was that despite a stringent control of the human experimental subjects, considerable variation in caries experience occurred in each group. This agrees with general clinical experience of great variations between individuals (*e.g.*, family groups) with similar environments. It is also of interest that about one or two persons per thousand are completely caries-free at the age of naval recruits.

This variability suggests that at best the relationship between dental caries experience and dietary factors is not a simple cause-effect relation, although much evidence exists that many carbohydrates can be considered as cariogenic under some conditions. The variability presumably arises from a number of factors, some of which can be classified as hereditary factors.

The most obvious hereditary factors are the size, shape, and arrangement of teeth in the mouth, the amount and composition of the saliva, and the relation of the soft tissues to the teeth. Most of these factors would be related to self-cleansing and food retention characteristics, although salivary effects could be even more profound and involve such components as buffers, antibacterial agents, and enamel rehardening materials.

Variability not related to genetic factors also could arise from differences and changes in the oral microflora. This factor recently has received considerable interest in the work of Keyes *et al.* (29). The maturation of tooth surfaces after eruption is another source of variation, one of the most critical known factors being exposure to fluorides in the diet or water.

**Controllable Factors.** The above causes of variability (except fluride) are essentially innate and not subject to dietary control. The problem that remains is to determine how to minimize the potential cariogenic effects of most dietary carbohydrates. Generally, the problem seems to reduce itself to determining how foodstuffs can be kept from contact or be removed from the teeth and oral cavity as rapidly as possible.

Sufficient evidence now exists to show that sticky carbohydrate-rich foods should be removed from the human diet as much as possible. This action will require the listing of specific items after careful consideration of the evidence. Presumably, this should be done by approved health agencies. The restriction of cariogenic substances to mealtimes also requires emphasis.

The same carbohydrate in different physical forms may vary markedly in caries-producing activity. This situation suggests that manufacturers of foodstuffs consider the relation to potential cariogenicity in their formulation and processing methods. In general, methods are probably available for making this judgment. Thus, Volker (33) made a preliminary study of an Army Field Ration and showed slow oral clearance.

In some instances, it may be possible also to substitute a less cariogenic for a more cariogenic component. Mixtures often are used widely in processed foods, but the judgment is mainly on taste and consistency, and not on cariogenicity. An alternative, possible in some applications, would be to incorporate cariostatic agents.

The accumulated scientific knowledge is currently such that the cariogenicity of carbohydrate products can be evaluated reasonably well. We now should be able to terminate the period in which most of the dental profession condemned carbohydrates of all types in all applications, and the food industry as a whole responded by refusals to consider the possible cariogenicity of its products. By cooperation of dental and health agencies with a receptive industry, dental caries experience can be reduced greatly.

### *Acknowledgment*

The preparation of this section was supported by a grant from the American Chicle Co., Division of Warner-Lambert Pharmaceutical Co. I also express my thanks to J. M. Navia for help in revising this manuscript.

### *Literature Cited*

(1) Bibby, B. G., Shaw, J. H., *Intern. Dental J.* **1965,** 15, 1.
(2) Blix, G. (Ed.), "Nutrition and Caries Prevention," Swedish Nutrition Foundation, Almqvist and Wiskells, Uppsala, 1965.
(3) Bowen, W. H., Cornick, D. E., *Helv. Odontol. Acta* **1967**, 11, 27.
(4) Brislin, J. F., Cox, G. J., "Survey of the Literature of Dental Caries," Univ. of Pittsburgh Press, Pittsburgh, Pa., 1964.
(5) Caldwell, R. C., *J. Dental Res.* **1962**, 41, 821.
(6) Caldwell, R. C., Bibby, B. G., *J. Dental Assoc.* **1958,** 57, 685.
(7) Csaky, T. Z., *Ann. N. Y. Acad. Sci.* **1965,** 131, 868.
(8) Frostell, G., Keyes, P. H., Larson, R. H., *J. Nutr.* **1967,** 93, 65.
(9) Gibbons, R. J., Socransky, S. S., *Arch. Oral Biol.* **1962,** 7, 73.
(10) Green, R. M., Hartles, R. L., *Arch. Oral Biol.* **1969,** 14, 235.
(11) Guggenheim, B., Konig, K. G., Herzog, E., Muhlemann, H. R., *Helv. Odontol. Acta* **1966,** 10, 101.
(12) Gustafson, G., Stellings, E., Abramson, E., Brumius, E., *Odontol. Tidskr.* **1953**, 61, 386.
(13) Haldi, J., Law, M. L., John, J., *J. Dental Res.* **1967,** 46, 739.
(14) Hall, H. D., Schneyer, C. A., *Proc. Soc. Exptl. Biol. Med.* **1964,** 117, 789.
(15) Halloway, P. J., Shaw, J. H., Sweeney, J., *Arch. Oral Biol.* **1961,** 3, 185.
(16) Koulourides, T., *Alabama Dental Rev.* **1963,** 11, 10.
(17) Krasse, B., *Arch. Oral Biol.* **1965,** 10, 215, 223.
(18) Lanke, L. S., *Acta Odontol. Scand.* **1957,** 15, Suppl. 23.

(19) Larson, R. H., *J. Am. Dietet. Assoc.* **1964**, 44, 368.
(20) Lundqvist, C., *Odontol. Rev.* **1952**, 3, Suppl. 1.
(21) Neumann, H. H., DiSalvo, N. A., *Ann. N. Y. Acad. Sci.* **1965**, 131, 893.
(22) Newbrun, E., *J. Dentistry Children* **1969**, 36, 239.
(23) Pigman, W., "The Carbohydrates," p. 807, Academic Press, New York, 1957.
(24) Pigman, W., *J. Am. Dental Assoc.* **1955**, 51, 685.
(25) Pigman, W., Brasher, J., Koulourides, T., *Nature* **1962**, 195, 190.
(26) Shaw, J. H., Griffiths, D., *J. Nutr.* **1963**, 80, 123.
(27) Shaw, J. H., Krumins, I., Gibbons, R. J., *Arch. Oral Biol.* **1967**, 12, 755.
(28) Sognnaes, R. F., Ed., "Advances in Experimental Caries Research," American Association for the Advancement of Science, Washington, D. C., 1955.
(29) Sognnaes, R. F., Ed., "Chemistry and Prevention of Dental Caries," Thomas, Springfield, Ill., 1962.
(30) Sognnaes, R. F., *J. Am. Dental Assoc.* **1948**, 37, 676.
(31) Stephan, R. M., *J. Dental Res.* **1966**, 45, 1551.
(32) Vipeholm Dental Caries Study, *Acta Odontol. Scand.* **1954**, 11, 195–388.
(33) Volker, J. F., *J. Am. Dental Assoc.* **1955**, 51, 285.
(34) Volker, J. F., "A Symposium on Preventive Dentistry," M. K. Hine, J. C. Muhler, Eds., Mosby, St. Louis, Mo., 1956.
(35) Volker, J. F., Caldwell, R. C., "Clinical Pedodontics," S. F. Finn, Ed., Saunders, Philadelphia, Pa., 1967.

RECEIVED August 14, 1968.

# 3

# Amino Acids, Proteins, and Dental Caries

ABRAHAM E. NIZEL

School of Dental Medicine, Tufts University, Boston, Mass. 02111

*Amino acids and proteins have the potential of being classified as anti-caries nutrients, like fluorides and phosphates. Animal and* in vitro *studies clearly show that natural protein foods like fish flour, purified compounds like casein, or amino acids like glycine have significant caries-inhibitory and cariostatic effects. The major question that needs to be resolved is whether these findings can be extrapolated to man. Also, we need to determine and understand the mechanisms responsible for producing this effect. It is conceivable that enrichment of sugar and sugar products with amino acids or protein concentrates to reduce their cariogenicity may soon be a reality if we expend more research efforts in this direction.*

On the basis of data obtained from *in vitro* studies and animal-feeding experiments, it appears that amino acids and dietary proteins may have an effect on dental caries development. However, in human subjects, a direct cause and effect relationship between protein and dental caries has yet to be demonstrated. Furthermore, very few of the studies reviewed in this section suggest the mechanism by which proteins and amino acids influence caries development. Both the lack of clinical studies and paucity of animal or *in vitro* experiments which deal with possible mechanisms of action indicate the urgent need for more research in protein–dental caries relationship, so that the full potential of protein as an anti-caries nutrient for the human may be realized.

### *Influence of Protein on Dental Caries in Human Beings*

**Population Studies.** Ockerse (29) noted that dental caries developed in only 20% of the children who were raised in the Northwest Cape Section of South Africa, an area where the intake of both dietary protein and fluoride are relatively high. This was in sharp contrast to a

100% incidence of caries found in children native to the Southern Region of the Cape, a region where the intake of protein and fluorides was correspondingly lower.

To substantiate his impression that protein foods and fluorides were related to this finding of lower caries incidence, Ockerse conducted an animal-feeding experiment in which female albino rats were fed during gestation and lactation one of the following diets: (1) control diet, (2) high carbohydrate–low protein diet, (3) low carbohydrate–high protein diet, (4) control diet plus 100 ppm F in water, and (5) low carbohydrate–high protein diet plus 100 ppm F in water. At 35 days of age, all the offspring were changed to a coarse corn diet, and continued on it for 45 days more. The mean caries index for each group was (1) 5.7; (2) 8.8; (3) 3.0; (4) 2.8; (5) 1.3. Thus, high carbohydrate and low fluorine intakes resulted in higher caries, while high protein and high fluorine intakes resulted in lower caries.

**Clinical Studies.** Attempts have been made by independent investigators to correlate the level of protein in the sera and saliva of humans with their dental caries experience. For example, Shannon and Gibson (*35*) measured the total protein, albumin, and globulin levels in the sera of 505 randomly-selected healthy young men. They were fed a ration which was adequate in all required nutrients. No correlations between caries incidence and the levels of total protein, albumin, and globulin in the sera were found.

Mandel *et al.* (*18*) studied a group of 63 caries-immune adults with a comparable group of caries-active adults by analyzing parotid saliva for content of total protein and protein-bound hexosamine and by comparing the distribution of various protein fractions and the ratios of fucose and hexosamine to nitrogen in the two major carbohydrate-proteins. No differences were found.

Stack (*39*) could find no correlation between the levels of salivary tryptophan and the DMF indices of 55 patients, even though such a correlation had been suggested by an earlier report of Turner and Crowell (*44*).

### *Influence of Natural Food Protein on Animal Caries*

**Cereals.** McClure (*22*) compounded diets containing 80% cereals which had been either heat-processed, cooked, or dried at 100°C., and fed them to rats, who developed smooth-surface caries. Since these finely pulverized diets were low in sugar content, he concluded that the cariogenicity of this diet was related to its low-quality protein content rather than the sugar.

In subsequent experiments, McClure (*20*) demonstrated a high incidence of smooth-surface caries in rats fed wheat flour, dry or toasted bread, or shredded wheat biscuit. When these cereal products were autoclaved in the presence of cerelose or starch, the caries potential was increased and supplements of 1% lysine counteracted this effect. He concluded that this amino acid (lysine) is the key cariostatic nutrient that is impaired during the processing or heating of cereals.

Dodds (*5*) was unable to confirm the report of McClure that heat-processing of cereals increases their cariogenicity, presumably because of reduced availability of their lysine content. She reported that rats fed diets composed mostly (80%) of either corn, rice, or oats developed smooth-surface caries, and that the relative cariogenicity of each of these cereals decreases as follows: wheat > corn > rice > oats.

**Dried Milk.** McClure and Folk (*24*) found that diets containing roller-processed skimmed milk powders were more cariogenic than spray-processed skimmed milk powders when fed in the diets of rats. Since higher temperatures are used in roller-processing than in spray-processing, and since lysine is partially inactivated when dry casein is heated, they concluded that the increased cariogenicity of the roller-dried milk probably was related to lysine impairment.

McClure and Folk (*23*) fed to rats diets in which the protein was supplied by three different nonfat milk powders (freeze-dried, spray-dried, and roller-dried), and they developed smooth-surface caries. The incidence of severity of the caries correlated with the degree of heat processing. Least caries developed in the group fed the freeze-dried milk and the most severe caries in the group fed the roller-dried milk powder. They later (*25*) demonstrated that caries development can be reduced by the addition of lysine to this type of diet.

The effect of dry whole milk on experimental caries has also been studied by Mauron *et al.* (*19*), who found, contrary to McClure, that this source of dietary protein was not cariogenic, and that there was no relationship between the content of utilizable lysine and the cariogenic potency of milk-containing diets. Dreizen *et al.* (*6*) came to a similar conclusion, because in their animal-feeding experiment they found that dry whole milk fed at a 39% level in a cariogenic diet had no appreciable effect on increasing cariogenicity.

Recently, Green (*10*) suggested that the cariogenicity of skimmed milk powder was related to its stickiness and the frequency with which it was eaten. Natural skimmed milk powder had a pleasanter taste than casein or a casein-rich simulated skimmed milk powder, and therefore was preferentially selected and eaten more frequently. All three diets (natural skimmed milk powder, casein, casein-rich simulated skimmed milk

### *Influence of Individual Amino Acid Supplements on Animal Caries*

**Lysine.** McClure (*22*) found that heat treatment caused an increase in cariogenicity of cereals, presumably because the availability of heat-labile lysine was decreased. McClure and Folk (*25*) later showed that the addition of L-lysine at levels of 2.5 and 0.25% to two cariogenic diets reduced the caries score in the rats significantly. Similarly, Bavetta and McClure (*1*) confirmed the cariostatic properties of lysine when they fed a cariogenic diet containing a considerable proportion of roller-processed skimmed milk powder to one group of rats, and fed the same diet supplemented with 0.4% lysine to a second group. The lysine supplement significantly retarded caries development, indicating that under these experimental conditions, lysine exerted a significant cariostatic action.

In an attempt to determine whether this action of lysine was local or systemic, McClure (*21*) designed an experiment in which lysine was administered in the diet, in the water, by intubation, or by intraperitoneal injection. Significant reduction in caries occurred when L-lysine was administered by diet, by water, and by intubation. Intraperitoneal injection had a variable and essentially negligible effect.

McClure (*20*) later reported a high incidence of smooth-surface caries in rats fed wheat flour, dry bread, toasted bread, or shredded wheat biscuit. When these cereal products were autoclaved in the presence of cerelose or starch, the caries potential was increased. Supplements of 1% lysine counteracted this effect.

Hennon (*12*) found that a lysine-deficient diet fed to rats under his experimental conditions produced the highest caries scores. Sharpenak *et al.* (*36*) showed that the addition of DL-lysine HCl to a caries-producing diet caused a decrease of approximately 50% in the number of carious teeth per rat, in the percentage of carious teeth, and in the caries index.

On the other hand, Dodds (*5*) reported that L-lysine HCl added to a cariogenic diet of raw whole wheat had no cariostatic effect.

**L-Arginine, L-Histidine, L-Ornithine, L-Cadaverine.** McClure and Folk (*23*) have reported that 0.5% L-arginine, 1% L-histidine, and 0.25% L-ornithine and L-cadaverine decreased caries development in rats fed an autoclaved skimmed milk powder diet.

**DL-Methionine and DL-Threonine.** Dodds (*5*) has reported that supplementation of DL-methionine and DL-threonine to a raw whole wheat cariogenic diet did not affect the incidence of caries.

**Glycine.** According to Dodds (*5*), the addition of 1.6% glycine to a white flour (wheat) cariogenic diet reduced the caries score by about 23.8%. Furthermore, when 0.20% of the glycine was replaced by 0.40% DL-methionine, the caries score was increased.

Harris *et al.* (*11*) also found that 4% glycine supplements could exert significant cariostatic activity when added to an otherwise cariogenic diet and fed to rats. In two successive feeding trials, caries was reduced by 66 and 43% by the 4% glycine dietary supplement.

**L-Glutamic Acid and L-Aspartic Acid.** Englander *et al.* (*8*) recently reported that neither L-glutamic acid nor L-aspartic acid influenced the development of caries in hamsters when added to a diet at a 2% level. These hamsters had been made highly susceptible to caries by oral swabbing with virulent cariogenic streptococci. The diet was rich in quality protein, was not deficient in lysine, and contained about 65% sucrose.

### *Protein and Bacteria Associated with Dental Caries Relationships*

Since dental caries is acknowledged to be a complex disease in which the metabolism of plaque bacteria play a significant role, the nutritional requirements of the oral microflora, especially their protein and amino acid needs, could be quite an important consideration here. The major proteinaceous constituent of saliva is the glycoprotein, mucin, and according to Leach's postulate (*15*) concerning the chemistry of dental plaque, the protein that is split from the glycoprotein by neuriminidase could contribute to the formation of plaque matrix. According to Loesche and Gibbons (*16*), the total quantity of amino acids is below the amount necessary for maximal growth of micro-organisms, but since bacteria in the mouth grow slowly and divide only a few times each day, this amount is of significance to the nutriture of the organisms. Unfortunately, there is very little more detailed information about the role of protein on cariogenic bacteria, with the exception of the following three studies.

Dreizen and Spies (*7*) investigated the products of protein putrefaction in saliva to determine whether some of them might be responsible for the decreased incidence of caries commonly seen in malnourished populations. They observed that indole and indole-3-acetic acid (which may be produced by the bacterial decomposition of tryptophan) decreased acid production and interfered with maximum growth of a strain of lactobacillus acidophilus found in the carious lesions.

Nordh (*27*) compared the serum protein patterns of two groups of people who had different numbers of lactobacilli in the saliva. The group with a high count (over 1 million/ml of saliva), which is associated with high caries activity, showed electrophoretic patterns in the serum, similar to those seen in inflammatory disease—i.e., decreased albumin, increased gamma globulin, and increased immunoglobulin concentrations.

Green (*9*) has suggested that innate caries resistance in people may be due to the presence of a bacteriolytic agent in the globulin fraction of the saliva. He claimed that this agent, which contains tryptophan and several related compounds, will reduce the growth of caries-promoting bacteria (lactobacilli and streptococci).

### *Effect of Protein and Amino Acids on Tooth Solubility*

Interesting *in vitro* studies of the effects of amino acids upon the rate of enamel and dentine solubilization when added to decalcifying buffers have been conducted at the Eastman Dental Center during recent years. Buonocore and Somner (*3*) compared aspartic acid, glutamic acid, alanine, and valine, and reported that aspartic acid was the most active in reducing the solubility of enamel in the presence of acetic, lactic, citric, and pyruvic acids, which are the organic acids commonly found in dental plaque and on enamel surfaces. This result suggested the possibility that the aspartic ion may function to reduce the rate at which these acids dissolve the tooth structure.

In subsequent studies, Koulourides and Buonocore (*14*) and Buonocore (*2*) found lysine to be an effective agent in reducing the rate of enamel decalcification. They postulated that surface-bond complexes are formed between amino acids and the enamel particles, and that these act to retard the diffusion of acids.

Significant reductions in enamel solubility were noted by Weiss and Bibby (*45, 46*) when casein solutions were added to decalcifying buffers. Milk protein concentrates were at least as good as whole milk in reducing enamel solubility. This result may indicate that neither the fat nor the mineral in the milk contribute to the reduction in enamel solubility. The importance of protein to this process was emphasized when these authors demonstrated that mucoproteins, such as gastric mucin, were equally as effective.

More recently, Pearce and Bibby (*31*) reported that enamel absorbs protein, and suggested that protein binding occurs in areas where enamel destruction is initiated. Thus, they demonstrated that there is a reaction between protein and the enamel surface. At the beginning of caries development (the white spot stage), decalcification is greater below the tooth surface than at the surface. Possibly this is because proteins cannot diffuse to subsurface sites.

### *Summary and Conclusions*

(1) It appears that both the amount and quality of protein are important factors in influencing dental caries development in the experimental animal. For example, Dodds noted less caries when the level of cereal protein was raised about 16% and when the diets were less deficient in amino acids. A diet which contains limited amounts of poor-quality protein will become less cariogenic as the protein content is increased, and/or as the quality of the protein is improved.

(2) Dietary additions of casein, a phosphoprotein, appeared to be the most effective of all proteins tested in the reduction of caries development in experimental animals. The relative importance of the phosphate moiety of the casein molecule for exerting this cariostatic action has not been evaluated.

(3) Other proteins and amino acids that show some promise as significant cariostatic agents are fish protein concentrate (F.P.C.) and glycine.

(4) A few *in vitro* studies seem to show that amino acids can decrease the rate of enamel solubility.

(5) No well-controlled study has been published which proves that dietary supplements of protein can influence the development of dental caries in human beings.

(6) The favorable indications that proteins and constituent amino acids may affect caries development should stimulate further search for protein-caries relationships.

### *Literature Cited*

(1) Bavetta, L. A., McClure, F., *J. Nutr.* **1957,** 63, 107.
(2) Buonocore, M. G., *J. Dent. Res.* **1963,** 42, 700.
(3) Buonocore, M. G., Somner, B., *J. Am. Dent. Assoc.* **1957,** 55, 781.
(4) Buxbaum, J. D., Kolin, H., Proutt, L. M., Osler, R. H., *J. Dent. Res.* **1957,** 36, 173.
(5) Dodds, M. L., *J. Nutr.* **1964,** 82, 217.
(6) Dreizen, S., Dreizen, J., Stone, R. E., *J. Dent. Res.* **1961,** 40, 1025.
(7) Dreizen, S., Spies, T. D., *J. Dent. Res.* **1947,** 26, 409.
(8) Englander, H. R., Keyes, P. H., Fitzgerald, R. J., *Arch. Oral Biol.* **1965,** 10, 599.
(9) Green, G. E., *J. Dent. Res.* **1959,** 38, 362.
(10) Green, R. M., *Helv. Odont. Acta* **1967,** 11, 32.
(11) Harris, R. S., Nizel, A. E., Navia, J. M., Das, S. K., *I.A.D.R. Abstracts,* March, 1967.
(12) Hennon, D. K., *J. Dent. Res.* **1960,** 39, 681.
(13) Holloway, P. J., Shaw, J. H., Sweeney, E. A., *Arch. Oral Biol.* **1961,** 3, 185.
(14) Koulourides, T. A., Buonocore, M. G., *J. Dent. Res.* **1961,** 40, 578.
(15) Leach, S. A., *Brit. Dent. J.* **1967,** 122, 537.
(16) Loesch, W. J., Gibbons, R. J., "Influence of Nutrition on the Ecology and Cariogenicity of the Oral Microflora" in Nizel, A. E., "The Science of Nutrition and its Application in Clinical Dentistry," W. B. Saunders Co., Philadelphia, Pa., 1966.
(17) Losee, F. L., VanReen, R., *J. Dent. Res.* **1957,** 36, 904-910.

(18) Mandel, S. D., Zorn, M., Ruiz, R., Thompson, R. H., Ellison, S. A., *Arch. Oral Biol.* **1965,** 10, 471.
(19) Mauron, J., Kinkel, H. J., Cremer, H. D., *Intern. J. Vitaminforsch.* **1959,** 30, 19.
(20) McClure, F. J., *J. Nutr.* **1958,** 65, 619.
(21) McClure, F. J., *Proc. Soc. Exptl. Biol. Med.* **1957,** 96, 631.
(22) McClure, F. J., *Science* **1952,** 116, 229.
(23) McClure, F. J., Folk, J. E., *J. Nutr.* **1955,** 55, 589.
(24) McClure, F. J., Folk, J. E., *Proc. Soc. Exptl. Biol. Med.* **1953,** 83, 21.
(25) McClure, F. J., Folk, J. E., *Science* **1955,** 122, 557.
(26) Nizel, A. E., King, G., Harris, R. S., Navia, J., I.A.D.R. Abstract #100, 1969.
(27) Nordh, F., *Acta Odont. Scand.* **1965,** 23, 187.
(28) Onisi, Ozaki, Hamada, *Japan. J. Dent. Health* **1966,** 16, 85.
(29) Ockerse, T. S., *African Dent. J.* **1941,** 15, 353.
(30) Osborn, M. O., Carey, J. F., Fisken, A. K., *J. Dent. Res.* **1966,** 45, 1564.
(31) Pearce, E. J. F., Bibby, B. G., *Arch. Oral Biol.* **1966,** 11, 329.
(32) Russell, A. L., White, C. L., *J. Dent. Res.* **1961,** 40, 594.
(33) Schweigert, B. S., Potts, E., Shaw, J. H., Zepplin, M., Phillips, P. H., *J. Nutr.* **1946,** 32, 405.
(34) Schweigert, B. S., Shaw, J. H., Zepplin, M., Elvehyem, C. A., *J. Nutr.* **1946,** 31, 439.
(35) Shannon, J. L., Gibson, W. A., *Oral Surg.* **1964,** 18, 399.
(36) Shapernak, A. E., Bobyleva, V. R., Gorozanina, L. A., *Vop. Piton* **1963,** 22, 239-244 (Kaf, bohin. Med. stomatol. Inst. Moscow) Russia.
(37) Shaw, J. H., *J. Nutr.* **1950,** 41, 1.
(38) Shaw, J. H., *J. Dent. Res.* **1966,** 45, 1810.
(39) Stack, M. V., *J. Dent. Res.* **1954,** 33, 316.
(40) Stephan, R. M., I.A.D.R. Abstract #365, 1968.
(41) Stephan, R. M., I.A.D.R. Abstract **1956,** 34, 77.
(42) Sweeney, E. A., Guzman, M., *Arch. Oral Biol.* **1966,** 11, 687.
(43) Tamura, S., Kizu, K., Ito, H., Nahai, K., *Bull. Tokyo Dent. Coll.* **1965,** 6, 15.
(44) Turner, N. D., Crowell, G. E., *J. Dent. Res.* **1947,** 26, 99.
(45) Weiss, M. E., Bibby, B. G., *Arch. Oral Biol.* **1966,** 11, 59.
(46) Weiss, M., Bibby, B. G., *Arch. Oral Biol.* **1965,** 10, 49.

RECEIVED August 15, 1968.

4

# Vitamins and Dental Caries

SAMUEL DREIZEN

University of Texas Dental Science Institute at Houston, Houston, Tex. 77025

*Vitamins contribute to both the pathogenesis and prevention of dental caries. During the formative period, vitamins A, C, and D are essential for proper deposition and calcification of tooth structure. Posteruptively, the vitamin–dental caries relationship is mediated primarily through the oral acidogenic microorganisms. The B vitamins nicotinic acid, pantothenic acid, and biotin are necessary growth factors for most if not all of the oral acidogenic flora. Some strains also require an exogenous source of thiamine and riboflavin. As components of the coenzymes which participate in anaerobic glycolysis, thiamine and nicotinic acid promote acid production by microbial action on locally retained ingested carbohydrates. Unfortunately, none of the B vitamins can be deleted safely from the diet for caries prevention without impairment of human health.*

The vitamins are a group of diverse organic compounds which are dietary in origin and indispensable for human health and well being. Most function as integral parts of enzyme systems involved in essential metabolic processes. As such, they are required in relatively small amounts in sharp contrast to the dietary macro-nutrients which contribute primarily to the structural makeup of cells and tissues.

Dental caries is a posteruptive disease of the teeth resulting from the action of cariogenic oral microorganisms on susceptible tooth structure in the presence of a suitable substrate and a favorable local environment. Various vitamins have been associated with the pathogenesis and prevention of dental caries. Some are caries-conducive; others caries-deterrent. Some affect the caries process by their presence; others by their absence. Some have a preeruptive influence which is exerted on the size, shape, and structure of the teeth. Others operate posteruptively by influencing the quantity and composition of the saliva and the makeup of the oral microbial flora. Evidence of the vitamin–dental caries relationship is detailed in this report.

### *Vitamin A*

**Effects of Deficiency.** Lack of vitamin A will produce characteristic abnormalities in the shape and structure of developing teeth, provided the deficiency is chronic enough and severe enough. The effects are mediated through alterations in the highly specialized odontogenic epithelium leading to disturbances in histo- and morphodifferentiation. In the rat, avitaminosis A induces enamel hypoplasia, irregular and atypical dentin formation, and epithelial invasion of the dental pulp (*79*). In man the primary histopathology is a metaplasia of the enamel-forming cells and an atrophy of the enamel organ which is manifested clinically as enamel hypoplasia (*11, 23*). Avitaminosis A is a rare cause of enamel hypoplasia in the human, since deficiencies of the degree and duration required to produce detectable dental defects are usually not compatible with life. Bloch (*10*) studied 64 blind Danish children with gross evidence of severe vitamin A deficiency during infancy and found neither conspicuous abnormalities in the form, position, and consistency of the teeth nor an increased predisposition to dental caries. Similarly, Shourie (*85*) found no greater incidence of dental caries in Indian children with skin and eye lesions suggestive of vitamin A deficiency than in adequately nourished ethnically identical children.

Paynter and Grainger (*71*) successfully modified the genetic template of tooth morphology by restricting pregnant rats to a synthetic diet deficient in vitamin A during the time the molar teeth were being formed in the offspring. The procedure caused the development of small molar teeth in the young to a degree which exceeded the range of normal variation. The size differences were not accompanied by gross tooth surface defects, severe histologic changes, metabolic derangements, or an increased caries susceptibility.

The only evidence of a direct relationship between dental caries and chronic vitamin A deficiency is supplied by Salley, Bryson, and Eshleman (*76*), who obtained a significant increase in caries in hamsters given a synthetic diet devoid of vitamin A. The caries-promoting potential of vitamin A deficiency was ascribed to a greatly reduced salivary flow precipitated by the deficiency related loss of secretory acini in the major and minor salivary glands. Xerostomia attributable to a keratinizing metaplasia and inflammatory reaction in both the salivary gland acini and ducts has been described in human vitamin A deficiency (*4*). Unfortunately, details of the cariogenicity of the xerostomia in these cases are lacking.

**Effects of Excess.** Dietary supplements of vitamin A neither stimulate nor suppress the caries tendency in children (*21, 64*). In a study by Day and Sedwick (*21*) at least 6000 U.S.P. units of vitamin A ingested daily in tablet form together with added vitamin D for 15 months not only failed to have a beneficial effect on the caries incidence, but afforded no measurable protection to the newly erupted teeth. In rats, addition of excessive amounts of water-soluble and fat-soluble vitamins including vitamin A did not alter significantly either the average number or average extent of carious lesions in animals whose tooth development was almost complete when the supplements were initiated (*82*).

### *Thiamine (Vitamin $B_1$)*

**Effects of Deficiency.** In 1958 Sharpenak (*81*) revived an hypothesis that a deficiency of cocarboxylase (thiamine pyrophosphate or diphosphothiamine) is an important cause of dental caries because of an accumulation of pyruvic acid in the dental and body tissues. This concept lacks supportive evidence and is in direct conflict with studies by Russell (*75*) in South Vietnam and Thailand and by Afonsky (*2*) in central China. They show that consumption of a nutritionally inadequate traditional diet, low or deficient in thiamine, is wholly compatible with a low caries prevalence.

**Effects of Excess.** Goll (*34*) tested the supposition that thiamine deficiency may be an etiologic factor in dental caries by feeding cakes prepared from thiamine-rich ingredients to a small group of German children. The thiamine intake per child was thus increased by 0.8 mg per day. No reduction in caries incidence was noted in the 9-month period of supplementation. Agapova (*3*) obtained a decrease in the dental caries attack rate in some of 75 children given a dietary additive of 2 mg thiamine daily for 2 years. The decrease was attributed to the suppressive action of thiamine on the cariogenic microorganisms. Thiamine has been found to be bacteriostatic when added to saliva *in vitro* at a level of 200 $\mu$grams per ml., a concentration which far exceeds the 0.2 to 1.4 $\mu$grams per 100 ml. normally present in human saliva (*8, 30*). In contrast, when present at a level of 2 $\mu$grams per ml. in a chemically defined complete synthetic medium, thiamine is growth-promoting rather than bacteriostatic for some strains of oral acidogens (*25*).

### *Riboflavin (Vitamin $B_2$)*

**Effects of Deficiency.** As shown by dental surveys in the United States (*55*), Guatemala (*46*), Nigeria (*91*), South Vietnam and Thailand (*75*), a diet deficient in riboflavin is not necessarily conducive to dental decay. Subjects with substandard riboflavin intakes and clinical evidence of the deficiency state were found to have a caries prevalence which was no higher and often much lower than in nutritionally superior control groups in the same region. Although riboflavin is a nutritional essential for some strains of oral lactobacilli, most will tolerate a riboflavin-free synthetic medium which is complete in all other nutritional essentials (*25, 51*).

**Effects of Excess.** Inclusion of riboflavin in the diet of rats in amounts far in excess of their nutritional needs does not alter their susceptibility to dental caries (*82*). There have been no comparable studies on the human level.

### *Nicotinic Acid (Niacin)*

**Effects of Deficiency.** Reports from various parts of the world indicate that endemic pellagrins have a low incidence of dental caries (*19, 49, 74, 77*). There is considerable evidence that the low caries prevalence and the nicotinic acid deficiency productive of pellagra are interrelated rather than fortuitous. Nicotinic acid has proved to be an irreplaceable nutritional factor for the oral lactic acid–producing bacteria (*25, 51*). Nicotinic acid amide acts as the functional group of codehydrogenases I and II, enzymes necessary for converting fermentable carbohydrates to acid residues. Within physiologic limits, the amount of acid production in saliva–glucose mixtures, *in vitro,* is related directly to the nicotinic acid content of the saliva sample (*24*). Addition of antimetabolites of nicotinic acid to such mixtures completely inhibits acid formation (*25, 53*). Incorporation of a metabolic antagonist of nicotinic acid in an experimental cariogenic diet fed weanling rats for 150 days reduced the caries tendency in these animals significantly (*26*). Conversely, deletion of nicotinic acid from a nutritionally balanced caries-producing hamster diet resulted in a reduction in caries incidence to approximately half that of the control group (*68*).

**Effects of Excess.** Koser and Kasai (*52*) found that comparatively huge quantities of nicotinic acid of the order of 10,000 times the nutritional requirement will prevent completely the growth of nicotinic acid-dependent bacteria *in vitro.* Experimentally, excessive amounts of nicotinic acid and other B vitamins increase the caries incidence in hamsters (*32*) and do not influence caries susceptibility in rats (*82*). Although massive doses of nicotinic acid are being used presently in treating some cases of hypercholesteremia in man, there have been no reports of the effect of this therapy on the human dentition.

### *Pyridoxine (Vitamin $B_6$)*

**Effects of Deficiency.** The possibility of a relationship between pyridoxine and dental caries was advanced by Rinehart and Greenberg (*73*) who observed that monkeys maintained on long term pyridoxine-deficient diets develop extensive dental caries. The pyridoxine deficiency–dental caries axis was apparent only after a minimum of 2 years of exposure to the deficient diets, with little or no adverse dental effects noted during the first 24 study months. Strean and co-workers (*90*) restricted small groups of hamsters to a cariogenic diet with and without added pyridoxine (50 mg/100 grams diet) for 10 months and obtained a significant reduction in frequency and extent of caries in the pyridoxine-supplemented group. Later Strean *et al.* (*89*) subjected hamsters to cariogenic diets low in pyridoxine (0.5 ppm) and high in pyridoxine (10 ppm) for 7 months and found a significant pyridoxine-associated diminution in caries frequency for the lower teeth but not for the upper teeth. The distinction in the locale of caries protection was ascribed to differences in the pyridoxine content of the saliva in various parts of the mouth, but no chemical evidence was offered to support this contention.

**Effects of Excess.** The caries preventive potential of pyridoxine has been tested in animals and in man with equivocal results. Wynn, Haldi, and Law (*94*) included relatively large amounts of pyridoxine (up to 100 ppm) in a synthetic high sucrose diet originally adequate in pyridoxine content. The added pyridoxine failed to reduce the cariogenicity of the test diet when fed to rats of a caries-susceptible strain. In contrast, Steinman and Hardinge (*87*) attained a notable reduction in caries incidence when rats were given a ration representative of the typical American diet supplemented with pyridoxine to the extent of 16 mg per kg food.

In a small pilot study, Strean *et al.* (*89*) achieved a 40% reduction in new carious lesions in 14 children, 10 to 15 years old, given lozenges containing 3 mg pyridoxine thrice daily for 1 year. The reference group was comprised of 14 children given placebo lozenges. Cohen and Rubin (*18*) used an identical testing procedure in 120 test children and 129 control children, 11 to 14 years of age, for 1 year and reported a slight suppressive effect of the pyridoxine lozenges on dental caries. The difference between the caries attack rates in the pyridoxine and placebo groups was not, however, statistically significant.

In adults the effects of pyridoxine supplements on dental caries experience has been tested in pregnant women by Hillman, Cabaud, and Schenone (*45*). Starting with the 4th month of pregnancy, 198 randomly selected pregnant women were given 20 mg pyridoxine once daily in capsule form, 169 were given a total of 20 mg pyridoxine thrice daily in lozenge form, and 173 received placebo preparations and served as controls. Each regimen was followed until parturition. The group not given added pyridoxine had an average DMF increase of 1.42 compared with 1.22 for the capsule group and 0.89 for the lozenge group. The difference between the mean DMF increments of the control and capsule groups was not significant; that between the control and lozenge groups was significant.

Strean (*88*) attributes the caries-deterrent action of pyridoxine to an alteration of the oral flora from a predominantly homofermentative lactic acid–producing type to a prevalence of heterofermentative forms which produce less lactic acid and more volatile end products. Since homofermentative forms do not and heterofermentative forms do utilize pyridoxine, the addition of pyridoxine creates a competitive system which eventuates in suppressing the heavy acid producers. Partial support for this contention is supplied by Palazzo, Cobe, and Ploumis (*70*), who showed that addition of pyridoxine in concentrations ranging from 1:2000 to 1:200,000 to suitable media inhibits homofermentative strains of the oral flora and promotes growth of the heterofermentative types. Although pyridoxine has been shown to be bacteriostatic against some strains of oral microorganisms when added to saliva in a concentration of 20 mg per 100 ml (*8*), levels of 200 mg per 100 ml failed to affect acid production in incubated saliva–glucose mixtures (*28*). A proper evaluation of the role of pyridoxine in the caries process awaits more intensive microbiologic, chemical, and clinical investigation.

### *Other B Vitamins*

Other B vitamins with a potential role in the caries process are biotin, pantothenic acid, folic acid, and inositol. Biotin and pantothenic acid resemble nicotinic acid in that they are essential for the growth and acid production of oral lactobacilli, streptococci, staphylococci, and yeasts in pure and mixed culture (*25, 51*). Mäkilä (*54*) found that the mean folic acid content of resting whole saliva in edentulous denture wearers and patients with teeth largely destroyed by caries is almost three times greater than that in subjects with slight caries activity. It was concluded that either a high saliva folic acid level promotes the development of caries, or the caries-precipitating factor leads to an increase in saliva folic acid concentration. Significant caries reductions have been obtained in rats fed cariogenic sugar diets containing 0.01–0.1% inositol (*67*). Addition of 1.4% phosphorylated inositol to a bread–glucose rat diet decreased the incidence of dental caries by an average of 77% and the caries severity score by an average of 91% (*59*). Studies by McCann,

Brady, and Gillen (*58*) indicate that enamel may pick up phosphate from phosphorylated inositol by ion exchange and that the increase in enamel phosphate contributes to the anticaries effectiveness of this compound in rats.

### *Vitamin C (Ascorbic Acid)*

**Effects of Deficiency.** Evidence that vitamin C is essential for normal tooth development is derived from histologic changes in the continuously forming incisors of scorbutic guinea pigs. These range from disturbed histodifferentiation of the odontoblasts culminating in amorphous and irregular dentin formation to a cessation of dentin deposition and overcalcification of the predentin. Atrophic changes in the enamel epithelium may occur in the late stages giving rise to enamel hypoplasia (*13*). Boyle (*12*) studied deciduous and permanent tooth germs of scorbutic infants and found no abnormalities except for some small cysts and minute hemorrhages in a few specimens. Teeth from scorbutic adults show porotic dentin, pulpal hyperemia and edema, and altered secondary dentin formation (*93*).

Despite the structural changes associated with scurvy, Westin (*93*) was unable to demonstrate any relationship between vitamin C deficiency and dental caries in the guinea pig, monkey, or man, nor is there any significant correlation between the vitamin C content of human blood, saliva, or urine and dental caries activity (*15, 44, 80*). Nevertheless, Ott (*69*) maintains that dental caries can be equated with disturbed vitamin C metabolism but offers little clinical and no experimental evidence to substantiate this claim. Hanke (*39*) supplemented the diets of 323 children with a pint of orange juice and the juice of one lemon daily and obtained an auspicious reduction in the intensity of caries. Administration of 90 ml. of orange juice daily failed to sustain the reduced caries activity, casting some doubt on the specificity of a dental caries–vitamin C deficiency relationship.

**Effects of Excess.** Vitamin C has been shown to be caries-promoting, caries-neutral, and caries-preventing—the specific role varying with the particular investigator. Thus, Hafer (*38*) regards pharmacologically effective doses of vitamin C as cariogenic since the administration of such doses is followed in a few weeks by a rise in lactobacillus counts and by a fall in the neutralizing power of the saliva. When incorporated in cariogenic diets in amounts ranging from 0.5–2.5% of the daily ration, vitamin C is without measurable effect on caries in rats (*50*) and in hamsters (*35*). In children, Grandison, Stott, and Cruikshank (*36*) found no significant modification in the caries course of 20 children given 200 mg vitamin C daily for 2 years. Dierks (*22*) reported that daily doses of 100 mg vitamin C are protective against the secondary decay which forms around filling margins, as no such lesions developed in children given vitamin C for 1 year. The lack of a control group and the failure to influence primary caries limits the value and applicability of these findings.

### *Vitamin D*

**Effects of Deficiency.** The changes induced by a vitamin D deficiency during the formative period of the teeth vary with the experimental animal. In all vitamin D-dependent species, the first and most prominent deficiency change is a line of disturbed calcification in the dentin. In the severe cases this is followed by a retardation of dentin formation and a failure of calcification of the predentin. In the rat, enamel formation and calcification are unaffected by a vitamin D deficiency, but guinea pigs, dogs, and man may develop hypoplastic enamel (*40*). Mellanby (*61*) was the first to suggest that teeth with imperfections in the enamel surface are more susceptible to caries than teeth without such defects. This concept has been both supported (*9, 20, 63*) and refuted (*21, 86*), with Mühlemann (*65*) expressing the contemporary opinion that while structural irregularities and hypoplasia of the enamel *per se* do not seem to increase caries susceptibility, they do favor post-eruptive plaque adherence and possibly caries attack owing to increased roughness.

Whether rachitic children have a greater tendency to dental decay than nonrachitic children as has been proclaimed by some (*27, 29*) and disputed by others (*43, 84*) is still unresolved. Numerous studies by Mellanby (*62*) imply that an adequate vitamin D intake during the period of tooth formation in children is associated with a reduced caries incidence. Attempts to establish a relationship between dental caries and the vitamin D content of the diet have been unsuccessful (*95*). Direct evidence that hypoplasia is caused by a deficiency of vitamin D or that adequate vitamin D *per se* will prevent hypoplasia or reduce the incidence of dental caries is still lacking (*40*).

**Effects of Excess.** The use of vitamin D supplements to control dental caries is beclouded by an inconsistency of results and interpretations. Claims for a caries-preventive action of vitamin D range from unmitigated effectiveness regardless of age, diet, and form administered (*57*) to those tempered by such limitations as: (a) vitamin D produces a substantial decrease in the dental caries experience of children when given between 3 and 10 years of age but not when given between 11 and 16 years of age (*5*); (b) vitamin D is more beneficial against caries when added to a deficient diet than to a well balanced diet (*78*); (c) vitamin D decreases dental caries susceptibility only when administered during the formative period and not after a tooth has already erupted (*6*); (d) vitamin D is more effective against caries when taken as cod liver oil than as irradiated ergosterol (*56*). Aebi (*1*) reconciles studies showing a caries-deterrent action of vitamin D with those which failed to change the caries pattern (*14, 21, 33, 48*) by postulating that other factors in the caries picture may supplement or negate the influence of vitamin D. In a more prosaic vein, Shaw (*83*) ascribes the lack of effect of vitamin D to a lack of an existing deficiency in the subjects given the supplements. In contrast, Volker (*92*) suggests that the special benefits noted with cod liver oil as compared with other preparations of vitamin D could be explained by the local action of the fats contained therein rather than by the form of the vitamin D.

### *Vitamin E*

Vitamin E is essential for maintaining the enamel organ of the rat incisor. A deficiency leads to premature atrophy and edema of the papillary layer, depigmentation, hypoplasia, bizarre anatomic forms, retarded eruption rate, and cyst formation in the adjacent connective tissue (*66, 72*). The parenchyma of the salivary glands is replaced by fat cells and fibrous connective tissue (*66*). Because of its antioxidant capacity, vitamin E has been tested against sulcul caries in the rat. Levels up to 0.5% $\alpha$-tocopherol in the diet failed to inhibit either caries or the growth of selected cariogenic microorganisms (*47*).

### *Vitamin K*

Of all presently known vitamins, only vitamin K prevents acid formation when added to saliva–glucose mixtures *in vitro* (*28*). The antibacterial properties of natural and synthetic vitamin K stem from their quinone structure which acts as an enzyme poison and not from the vitamin activity (*7, 17*). The efficacy of vitamin K in controlling dental caries by inhibiting the enzymes involved in the microbial degradation of carbohydrates has been studied in rats, hamsters, and man.

In rats, prolonged administration of synthetic vitamin K in concentrations ranging from 0.005 to 0.8% of a cariogenic diet failed to exert a measurable effect on the caries incidence (*41*). In hamsters, vitamin K prevented dental decay when 1 mg was added to the diet every second day or when 1 mg was injected intraperitoneally every third day (*31*). In man, chewing a stick of gum containing 0.75 mg 2-methyl-1,4-naphthoquinone sodium bisulfite addition compound (synthetic vitamin K) for at least 10 minutes after each meal for a period of 18 months by 58 subjects reduced the development of new carious lesions by from 60 to 80% depending on the basis of comparison (*16*). The validity of these conclusions has been challenged by Shaw (*83*) who analyzed the data in the absence of a statistical evaluation by the authors and by a subsequent study in which chewing a synthetic vitamin K-containing gum after ingestion of food or drink had no caries-suppressive effect on clinical and radiographic examination (*60*).

### *Vitamin P*

Rutin, a compound with vitamin P-like activity, and hesperidin, an integral part of the vitamin P molecule, each with antioxidant properties, have been investigated for possible anticariogenic activity. Neither prevented caries in rats when incorporated in a caries-inducing diet nor inhibited the growth of selected bacteria usually encountered in the oral cavity. In a single trial in which rats were fed 0.5% hesperidin, there was actually a statistically significant increase in caries score (*47*).

### *Vitamin Mixtures*

**Effects of Deficiencies.** Green and Hartles (*37*) performed a series of short term experiments (20–21 days) designed to test the effect of multiple vitamin deletion on caries production without inducing frank deficiency states. Omission of all fat-soluble vitamins from a cariogenic diet was without effect on the caries experience of weanling albino rats, whereas an absence of all water-soluble vitamins resulted in a significant decrease in caries development. The latter was attributed, in part, to a diminished food intake and disturbed eating pattern since the rats failed to grow on the water-soluble vitamin deficient diet.

**Effects of Supplements.** The anticariogenic effectiveness of mixed vitamin preparations was investigated in a series of 436 healthy children ranging in age from birth to 5.5 years (*42*). Each received a daily dietary supplement of 3000 to 4000 units vitamin A, 400 units vitamin D, 60 to 75 mg vitamin C, 1.0 to 1.2 mg thiamine, 1.2 to 1.5 mg riboflavin, and 8 to 15 mg niacinamide for 36 months. This regimen failed to exert a measurable cariostatic action unless 0.5 to 1.0 mg fluoride as sodium fluoride was incorporated in the daily vitamin supplement.

### *Summary and Conclusions*

In the preeruptive period, vitamins A, C, and D are essential for the proper deposition and mineralization of tooth structure. Although well formed teeth are not necessarily synonymous with caries resistance, such teeth may provide fewer opportunities for plaque attachment, plaque retention, and caries activity.

In the posteruptive period, the vitamin–dental caries relationship is mediated primarily through the oral acidogenic flora. All cariogenic microorganisms are, to a certain extent, vitamin-dependent and require an exogenous supply of some or many of these nutrients. The spectrum of need varies with the particular organism. The B vitamins nicotinic acid, pantothenic acid, and biotin are necessary growth factors for most, if not all, lactic acid bacteria. Some strains also require thiamine, riboflavin, and folic acid. As components of the coenzymes involved in anaerobic glycolysis, thiamine and nicotinic acid facilitate the production of organic acids by microbial action on retained ingested carbohydrates.

Diets completely devoid of the vitamins which serve as essential growth factors for the oral acidogenic organisms or as glycolytic coenzyme components are caries-inhibitory. Unfortunately, these vitamins cannot be deleted safely from the diet without disastrous consequences to human health. Conversely, there is, as yet, no clear and uncontestable evidence that dietary supplements of any of the presently known vitamins is protective against human dental caries.

### *Literature Cited*

(1) Aebi, H., *Nutr. Dieta* **1964,** 5, 82.
(2) Afonsky, D., *J. Dental Res.* **1951,** 30, 53.
(3) Agapova, O. I., *Stomatologiya* **1954,** 33, 17.
(4) Allington, H. V., *Arch. Dermatol. Syphilis* **1950,** 62, 829.
(5) Anderson, P. G., Williams, C. H. M., Halderson, H., Summerfeldt, C., Agnew, R. G., *J. Am. Dental Assoc.* **1934,** 21, 1349.
(6) Armstrong, W. D., *J. Dental Res.* **1948,** 27, 376.
(7) Armstrong, W. D., Knutson, J. W., *Proc. Soc. Exptl. Biol. & Med.* **1943,** 52, 307.
(8) Balogh, K., Petrucz, K., Angyal, J., *J. Dental Res.* **1960,** 39, 886.
(9) Bibby, B. G., *J. Dental Res.* **1943,** 22, 218.
(10) Bloch, C. E., *Am. J. Diseases Children* **1931,** 42, 263.
(11) Boyle, P. E., *J. Dental Res.* **1933,** 13, 39.
(12) Boyle, P. E., *J. Dental Res.* **1934,** 14, 172.
(13) Boyle, P. E., Wolbach, S. B., Bessey, O. A., *J. Dental Res.* **1936,** 15, 331.
(14) Bruszt, P., *Oesterr. Z. Stomatol.* **1958,** 55, 72.
(15) Burrill, D. Y., *J. Dental Res.* **1942,** 21, 330.
(16) Burrill, D. Y., Calandra, J. C., Tilden, E. B., Fosdick, L. S., *J. Dental Res.* **1945,** 24, 273.
(17) Calandra, J. C., Fancher, O. E., Fosdick, L. S., *J. Dental Res.* **1944,** 23, 31.
(18) Cohen, A., Rubin, C., *Bull. Phila. County Dental Soc.* **1958,** 22, 84.
(19) Corkill, N. L., *Lancet* **1934,** 1, 1387.
(20) Davies, J. N., *Brit. Dental J.* **1939,** 67, 66.
(21) Day, C. D. M., Sedwick, H. J., *J. Nutr.* **1934,** 8, 309.
(22) Dierks, K., *Zahnaerztl. Rundschau.* **1943,** 52, 645.
(23) Dinnerman, M., *Oral Surg. Oral Med. Oral Pathol.* **1951,** 4, 1024.

(24) Dreizen, S., Reed, A. I., Spies, T. D., *Intern. Z. Vitaminforsch.* **1951**, 22, 396.
(25) Dreizen, S., Spies, T. D., *J. Dental Res.* **1953**, 32, 65.
(26) Dreizen, S., Spirakis, C. N., Stone, R. E., *Intern. Z. Vitaminforsch.* **1963**, 33, 321.
(27) Eliot, M. M., Souther, S. P., Anderson, B. G., Arnim, S. S., *Am. J. Diseases Children* **1934**, 48, 713.
(28) Fancher, O. E., Calandra, J. C., Fosdick, L. S., *J. Dental Res.* **1944**, 23, 23.
(29) Firu, P., Diaconescu, M., Cristea, M., Gherga-Negrea, A., Cristea, I., *Stomatologia (Bucharest)* **1965**, 12, 139.
(30) Fujishiro, I., *Igaku To Seibutsagaku* **1952**, 23, 59.
(31) Gebauer, H., *Deut. Zahnaerztl. Z.* **1955**, 10, 555.
(32) Gebauer, H., Plathner, C. H., *Deut. Zahnaerztl. Z.* **1959**, 14, 1693.
(33) Goll, H., *Wien. Klin. Wochenschr.* **1939**, 52, 35.
(34) Goll, H., *Med. Klin.* **1940**, 26, 712.
(35) Granados, H., Glavind, J., Dam, H., *J. Dental Res.* **1949**, 28, 670.
(36) Grandison, W. B., Stott, L. B., Cruikshank, D. B., *Brit. Dental J.* **1942**, 72, 237.
(37) Green, R. M., Hartles, R. L., *Arch. Oral Biol.* **1966**, 11, 913.
(38) Hafer, H., *J. Dentistry Belge* **1959**, 50, 187.
(39) Hanke, M. T., "Diet and Dental Health," p. 142, The University of Chicago Press, Chicago, 1933.
(40) Hartles, R. L., Slack, G. L., *Proc. Nutr. Soc.* **1959**, 18, 79.
(41) Hatton, E. H., Dodds, A., Hodge, H. C., Fosdick, L. S., *J. Dental Res.* **1945**, 24, 283.
(42) Hennon, D. K., Stookey, G. K., Muhler, J. C., *J. Dentistry Children* **1966**, 33, 3.
(43) Hess, A. F., Abramson, H., *Dental Cosmos* **1931**, 73, 849.
(44) Hess, W. C., Smith, B. T., *J. Dental Res.* **1949**, 28, 507.
(45) Hillman, R. W., Cabaud, P. G., Schenone, R. A., *Am. J. Clin. Nutr.* **1962**, 10, 512.
(46) Hurtate, A., Scrimshaw, N. S., *J. Dental Res.* **1955**, 34, 390.
(47) Jordan, H. V., Bowler, A. E., Berger, N. D., *J. Dental Res.* **1961**, 40, 878.
(48) Jundell, I., Hanson, R., Sandberg, T., *Acta Paediat.* **1938**, 23, 141.
(49) Kniesner, A. H., Mann, A. W., Spies, T. D., *J. Dental Res.* **1942**, 21, 259.
(50) Konig, K. G., Mühlemann, H. R., *Helv. Odontol. Acta* **1964**, 8, 72 suppl. 1.
(51) Koser, S. A., Fisher, B. J., *J. Dental Res.* **1950**, 29, 760.
(52) Koser, S. A., Kasai, G. J., *J. Bacteriol.* **1947**, 53, 743.
(53) Krasse, B., *Acta Odontol. Scand.* **1954**, 12, 173.
(54) Mäkilä, E., *Arch. Oral Biol.* **1966**, 11, 839.
(55) Mann, A. W., Dreizen, S., Spies, T. D., Hunt, F. M., *J. Am. Dental Assoc.* **1947**, 34, 244.
(56) McBeath, E. C., Verlin, W. A., *J. Am. Dental Assoc.* **1942**, 29, 1393.
(57) McBeath, E. C., Zucker, T. F., *J. Nutr.* **1938**, 15, 547.
(58) McCann, M. C., Brady, R. R., Gillen, W. R., *New Zealand Dental J.* **1962**, 58, 244.
(59) McClure, F. J., *J. Nutr.* **1960**, 72, 131.
(60) Medical Department Professional Service Schools, *Bull. U. S. Army Med. Dept.* **1946**, 5, 265.
(61) Mellanby, M., *Brit. Dental J.* **1923**, 44, 1.
(62) Mellanby, M., *Med. Res. Council, Spec. Repts. Ser. (London)* **1934**, 191.
(63) Mellanby, M., *Brit. Med. J.* **1940**, 1, 1341.
(64) Mellanby, M., Pattison, C. L., *Brit. Med. J.* **1928**, 2, 1079.
(65) Mühlemann, H. R., "Nutrition and Caries Prevention," G. Blix, Ed., p. 9, Almqvist and Wiksells, Upsalla, Sweden, 1965.

(66) Nelson, M. A., Jr., Chaudry, A. P., *J. Dental Res.* **1966,** 45, 1072.
(67) Novotny, J., *Cesk. Stomatol.* **1960,** 60, 350.
(68) Orland, F. J., Hemmens, E. S., Harrison, R. W., *J. Dental Res.* **1950,** 29, 512.
(69) Ott, E., *Int. Z. Vitaminforsch.* **1958,** 29, 83.
(70) Palazzo, A., Cobe, H. M., Ploumis, E., *N. Y. State Dental J.* **1959,** 25, 303.
(71) Paynter, K. J., Grainger, R. M., *J. Can. Dental Assoc.* **1956,** 22, 519.
(72) Pindborg, J. J., *J. Dental Res.* **1952,** 31, 805.
(73) Rinehart, J. F., Greenberg, L. D., *Am. J. Clin. Nutr.* **1956,** 4, 318.
(74) Roberts, S. R., "Pellagra," p. 109, C. V. Mosby Co., St. Louis, 1912.
(75) Russell, A. J., *J. Dental Res.* **1963,** 42, 233.
(76) Salley, J. J., Bryson, W. F., Eshleman, J. R., *J. Dental Res.* **1959,** 38, 1038.
(77) Sandwith, F. M., "The Medical Diseases of Egypt," p. 296, H. Kempton, London, 1905.
(78) Schoenthal, L., Brodsky, R. H., *Am. J. Diseases Children* **1933,** 46, 91.
(79) Schour, I., Massler, M., *Physiol. Rev.* **1945,** 25, 442.
(80) Shannon, I. L., Gibson, W. A., *Arch. Oral Biol.* **1964,** 9, 371.
(81) Sharpenak, A. E., *Stomatol. Moscow* **1958,** 37, 3.
(82) Shaw, J. H., *Proc. Soc. Exptl. Biol. & Med.* **1949,** 70, 479.
(83) Shaw, J. H., *Natl. Acad. Sci.—Natl. Res. Council* **1952,** Publ. 225, 415.
(84) Shelling, D. H., Anderson, G. M., *J. Am. Dental Assoc.* **1936,** 23, 840.
(85) Shourie, K. L., *Indian J. Med. Res.* **1942,** 30, 561.
(86) Staz, J., *S. African Med. J.* **1943,** 17, 1.
(87) Steinman, R. R., Hardinge, M. G., *J. Dental Res.* **1958,** 37, 874.
(88) Strean, L. P., *Schweiz. Monatsschr. Zahnheilk.* **1957,** 67, 981.
(89) Strean, L. P., Bell, F. T., Gilfillan, E. W., Emerson, G. A., Howe, E. E., *N. Y. State Dental J.* **1958,** 24, 133.
(90) Strean, L. P., Gilfillan, E. W., Emerson, G. A., *N. Y. State Dental J.* **1956,** 22, 325.
(91) Tabrah, F. L., *Science* **1962,** 138, 38.
(92) Volker, J. F., "A Symposium on Preventive Dentistry," J. C. Muhler and M. K. Hine, Eds., p. 45, The C. V. Mosby Co., St. Louis, 1956.
(93) Westin, G., *Dental Cosmos* **1925,** 67, 868.
(94) Wynn, W., Haldi, J., Law, M. L., *J. Nutr.* **1960,** 70, 69.
(95) Youmans, J. B., Patton, E. W., Sutton, W. R., Kern, R., Steinkamp, R., *Am. J. Public Health* **1944,** 34, 1049.


RECEIVED August 14, 1968.

# 5

# Antibiotics and Dental Caries

BASIL G. BIBBY

Eastman Dental Center, Rochester, N. Y. 14603

*When fed in water or diet, penicillin and some other antibiotics consistently limit caries activity in animals. Topical applications on animals' teeth seem to have some effect. Clinical studies in human subjects using antibiotics in dentifrices or as prophylaxis against rheumatic fever gave inconsistent results. While negative findings are probably related to the manner of use rather than the absence of inherent cariostatic properties, an important consideration is that long-range ill effects may result from disturbance of the ecological balance of the oral flora.*

The initial studies on the relationships between antibiotics and dental caries were designed to indicate the importance of bacteria or certain bacterial groups in its etiology. Thereafter, attempts were made to establish the usefulness of certain antibiotics in caries prevention in man. Recently they have been used again in caries research for evaluating the importance of specific bacterial types and testing new ideas in caries etiology.

Twenty years ago, the belief that gram positive bacteria, such as the streptococci, were the activating agents of dental decay was not as generally accepted as it is today, and some dental investigators believed that inadequate nutrition might have equal importance. One way of settling this question was to add an agent, such as penicillin, which would destroy acid-producing gram positive organisms, to a diet which was known to cause dental decay in rats, and see whether it would protect the animals against caries. In such an experiment, it was found (*29*) that rats eating a caries-producing diet with 75 units of penicillin per gram of food or water developed no dental decay, whereas animals eating the penicillin-free control diet developed caries as usual. The lactobacilli, which at that time were believed to be causative agents of caries, had been eliminated from the mouths of the penicillin group. Following this approach, Stephan *et al.* (*36, 37*) tested the effect of penicillin, Aureomycin, bacitracin, Chloromycetin, streptomycin, Terramycin, cephalosporin, and polymyxin on rat caries for the double purpose of determining the relative effectiveness of these agents in preventing caries and indicating which spectra of microorganisms played the most important part in its etiology. Their findings showed that only cephalosporin and polymyxin failed to reduce caries, and that none of the broad-spectrum antibiotics was any more effective than penicillin in this respect. The failure of cephalosporin, which is effective against most gram positive organisms except some streptococci and lactobacilli, to retard caries indicated the importance of these bacterial types in caries. The negative results with polymyxin likewise showed that gram negative organisms had no significance in the causation of rat caries.

Fitzgerald and Jordan (*5*) tested 10 units or 10 $\mu$g per gram of several different antibiotics in cariogenic diets in a rat study. All the agents significantly reduced the caries score below that given by the control diet. Penicillin was most effective, with only one third of the animals showing caries, followed in order by orythromycin, zinc bacitracin, carbomycin, and neomycin.

In a study of the mechanisms of caries prevention by various agents, McClure *et al.* (*28*) found that penicillin at 10 units per gram of diet was more effective in preventing caries in white rats than 50 ppm of sodium fluoride or iodoacetic acid or a high-mineral diet. They interpreted this to mean that bacterial activity on the teeth was of primary importance in causing caries.

In endeavoring to determine which types of bacteria produced caries in their caries-susceptible strain of rats, Rosen *et al.* (*33*) found that when 500 units of penicillin or 0.025% Terramycin per gram of diet were fed, no caries occurred in the penicillin rats, but all their Terramycin rats showed caries. Since both antibiotics are effective against gram positive organisms, they concluded that some unrecognized types of bacteria must be responsible for caries in their animals.

Shaw and Sweeney (*34*) used cotton rats, white rats, and desalivated white rats in a comparison of the effectiveness of different levels of a variety of antibiotic agents on caries, and also compared their *in vitro* effectiveness against a human and rat strain of *Lactobacillus acidophilus*. Penicillin was the most effective in reducing caries in both species. Aureomycin, Chloromycetin, streptomycin, and Terramycin were moderately effective, whereas panthenol, tyrothricin, subtilin, and bacitracin gave only slight or no protection. No correlation was found between effectiveness in reducing animal caries and the ability to prevent acid formation in the lactobacillus cultures. Falla and Shaw (*4*) showed that injected penicillin would reduce caries in rats, but to be effective, levels twice as high as in the food had to be used.

Using a 15-day, rather than the usual 80- to 100-day, experimental period, Muhlemann *et al.* (*31*) made an extensive comparison of dietary additions of 0.01 to 0.2% of antibacterial and antifungal antibiotics and other antibacterial chemical and cariostatic agents on the initiation of rat caries. The antibacterial agents used were penicillin, Aureomycin, Declomycin, erythromycin, Oleandomycin, novobiocin, thiostrepton, bacitracin, dihydrostreptomycin, and chloramphenicol. The antimycotic agents used were nystatin, griseofulvin, amphotericin B, echinomycin, usnic acid, and flavofungin. The antibiotics with gram positive spectra—penicillin, Oleandomycin, erythromycin, and novobiocin—were most effective in preventing early caries, and their briefly-presented results can be interpreted as showing caries reductions of from 85 to 90% below the water controls. Tetracyclines—Aureomycin, Tetracyn, and Declomycin—generally gave reductions in the 60% range and in this respect were comparable in effectiveness to sodium fluoride, as were the antibiotics with both gram positive and gram negative spectra. Neither the antimycotics nor the disinfectants reduced caries. From these results, it was concluded that the antibiotics were the most effective agents against rat caries.

The obvious conclusion from all of these studies is that antibiotics are capable of preventing dental decay in animals. Several of them are very potent, and their effectiveness seems to be related to the capacity to interfere with the growth of gram positive bacteria in general, rather than the lactobacilli in particular.

The demonstrated effectiveness of antibiotics in preventing animal caries led to a consideration of their use to combat dental decay in man. As a result, both *in vitro* and animal caries studies were undertaken, with a view to developing prophylactic products for human use.

The *in vitro* experiments were based on the knowledge that dental caries results from decalcification of teeth by acids formed by bacterial fermentation of carbohydrates, and, therefore, any agent which would effectively interfere with the production of acid would be likely to prevent tooth decay. Using this approach, large numbers of antibacterial agents and enzyme inhibitors have been tested in several ways to indicate their potential usefulness in preventing caries. Zander and Bibby (*44*) measured reduction of acid formation from glucose in saliva, Fosdick (*9*) calcium loss from enamel in a salivary fermentation system, and Mahler and Manly (*27*) acid formation in an "artificial plaque" composed of packed organisms obtained by centrifuging mouth washings. In our experiments, and Fosdick's, penicillin was the most effective of the many agents tested. Fosdick concluded that since penicillin was absorbed in protein films, and other enzyme inhibitors were not, it would have a lasting effect on the caries-producing activity of the bacterial plaques on the tooth surface. However, in Mahler and Manly's (*27*) experiments, in which packed microorganisms were used rather than suspensions, penicillin was ineffective in changing the course of acid production. This finding on short-term acid formation in "artificial plaque" was extended into the mouth by Brudevold and Hawes' (*3*) finding that penicillin did not interfere with acid formation in plaques on human tooth surfaces.

A different sort of *in vitro* evidence on the effectiveness of penicillin in preventing caries was offered by Zander and Bibby (*44*), who showed that saliva collected from human mouths 2 hours after a penicillin rinse still lacked the ability to ferment glucose.

While attention has been centered on penicillin, other antibiotics give comparable inhibition of acid formation in *in vitro* tests (*2, 29*). Brudevold and Bibby (*2*) found that among experimentally developed antibiotics that the manufacturers deemed unsuitable for systemic administration there were some which were equally as effective as penicillin in reducing acid production by mouth bacteria. From this, it may be suggested that the long-range possibilities of utilizing antibiotics in caries control might well depend upon the selection of types which would not be employed for any other medical purpose.

Several animal-feeding studies designed to supplement those already cited have been carried out to select and evaluate antibiotics for inclusion in dentifrices intended for caries prevention in man. Looking towards finding the lowest effective concentration of penicillin which would be effective against caries, Webman *et al.* (*40*) showed that as little as 2 units of penicillin added to a caries-producing diet reduced dental decay in rats by almost a third, and that a reduction of lactobacillus count and an increase of gram negative organisms also occurred in the animals' mouths. Volker *et al.* (*38*) compared the effect of penicillin, a mercuric benzoate, and a sarcosinate, all of which inhibited acid production by salivary bacteria and were retained on the tooth surface, on hamster caries. They found penicillin to be the most effective under the two test conditions used. In another comparison of the effectiveness of penicillin and other cariostatic agents, Pindborg (*32*) found that 20 mg of procaine penicillin per kg of diet (the equivalent of 20 international units per gram of diet) reduced dental decay by 81%, whereas 10 ppm of sodium fluoride or of stannous fluoride added to the same diet gave caries reductions of only 31.6 and 28.9, respectively.

Another type of experiment, in which antibiotic mixtures were brushed on animal teeth, has been used to predict the potential effectiveness of antibiotic dentifrices in man. In the first experiment of this sort, Zander and Bibby (*44*) brushed a solution containing 500 units of penicillin per cc on the teeth of hamsters which were kept on a caries-producing diet for 40 days. In eight animals whose teeth were brushed with penicillin, there was less than one cavity per animal, whereas in the water-brushed control group, the animals had an average of seven cavities. In another hamster experiment (*45*), solutions containing various concentrations of penicillin, Aureomycin, and tyrothricin were brushed on the teeth. Penicillin was most effective. To select a dentifrice for clinical testing in children, Shiere (*35*) brushed five different tyrothricin dentifrices and a control on hamster teeth. The one which gave the maximal caries reduction, 25.6% below the control, was subsequently found equally effective in man.

The accumulated evidence that penicillin would interfere with acid formation by salivary bacteria and would unquestionably prevent dental caries in animals led to tests of its caries-preventive effect in man.

Before mentioning the findings in the clinical tests which have been carried out using antibiotic dentifrices, it should be pointed out that many variables beyond that of the agent used complicate the obtaining of reliable results in human studies. For instance, an agent which is effective in animals may not be of any use in man, or one examination and recording procedure may fail to show differences which would appear if another were used, but most importantly, the whole result is going to depend upon the extent to which the instructions on the use of the test dentifrice are followed. Obviously, no therapeutic agent can be expected to produce benefit as long as it remains in its container.

Several clinical tests on the effect of antibiotic dentifrices on caries have been reported. The first study, that of Hill *et al.* (*15*), used a powder containing 500 units of penicillin per gram and produced no apparent reduction in dental decay, although a reduction in salivary lactobacillus count was observed. However, since the test subjects were 8- to 16-year-old boys whose unsupervised brushing habits are most unpredictable, the negative result could have been the result of limited use of the dentifrice. In another study, Zander (*43*) found a 55% reduction in dental decay in 6- to 14-year-old children in the first year, and a 57.6% reduction in the second year when a powder containing 500 units of penicillin per gram was brushed on the teeth under supervision five times per week in school. In the third test of an antibiotic dentifrice (*16*), 1000 units of penicillin per gram in an anhydrous creamy base was used under supervised brushing. It was only slightly effective in reducing dental decay and did not reduce the lactobacillus count in the saliva. The lack of success in this instance could have been caused by the penicillin not being liberated from the dentifrice rapidly enough in the mouth. In a small test (*39*) with a powder containing 100 units of penicillin per gram, orphanage children showed no slowing of the caries attack or reduction of the lactobacillus count as compared with the controls. In the only dentifrice study with an antibiotic other than penicillin (*35*), a tyrothricin dentifrice which had been shown to be effective against hamster caries gave a 26% reduction in dental decay when compared with a control paste.

Using only lactobacillus counts and acid formation by aciduric mouth organisms to assess caries activity, Ludwick *et al.* (*26*) compared different concentrations of several antibiotics and other agents over 6- to 7-week periods. They found that a powder containing 0.07% penicillin was more effective than powders containing tyrothricin, streptomycin, gramicidin, bacitracin, and other anticaries agents. The effect of an antibiotic in a mouthwash on caries seems to have been tested only once (*23*), in which a 1-year trial of bacitracin in a mouthwash failed to reduce caries. While penicillin has been incorporated into chewing gum and troches for other oral uses, there does not seem to have been any organized study of their effect on dental caries.

Reason for believing that penicillin is capable of reducing dental decay in human subjects has come from another type of use. Many children are placed on prophylactic penicillin for the control of rheumatic fever or as a means of combatting chronic pulmonary diseases. Several comparisons have been made of patients under such therapy. In one of these (*25*), rheumatic fever patients who had been on prophylactic penicillin from the age of 7 years had approximately 40% fewer carious teeth than children of comparable age without antibiotic experience. In a later study (*13*), 75 and 74 children who received daily oral penicillin, respectively, 200,000 units for the prevention of recurrent rheumatic fever and 1–3,000,000 units with occasional tetracycline for chronic respiratory diseases, showed only one third of the caries increment of control subjects.

The *in vitro* and animal studies, together with preliminary clinical evidence of caries reduction in man, resulted in the brief appearance on the market of two penicillin dentifrices. Several reasons contributed to their disappearance. One of these was that competing therapeutic dentifrices with greater cosmetic appeal were offered at about the same time. Another is that they were treated with suspicion by both the medical and dental professions, which, as experience grew, attached increasing weight to the dangers of developing penicillin-resistant organisms and allergic states. The evidence on this latter subject rests in some demonstrations that the mouths of children using penicillin dentifrices contained increased populations of gram negative organisms in two studies (*14, 42*). Children using Zander's 500-unit penicillin powder for 1½ years did not show an increase in penicillin-resistant lactobacilli (*8*) or streptococci and staphylococci (*22*), but after 3 years more penicillin-resistant streptococci, micrococci, and neisseria were found (*21, 41*). In patients on 200,000–3,000,000 units of oral penicillin per day, a slight increase in antibiotic resistance was noted without any significant change in bacterial ecology of the mouth (*11*). However, failure to establish the safety of penicillin in the face of indications of increases in the number of penicillin-resistant bacterial types resulted in unfavorable opinion from an Ad Hoc Committee of the Federal Food and Drug Administration (*24*), and likewise, the Council on Dental Therapeutics of the American Dental Association offered a critical opinion (*17*), recommending that "penicillin dentifrices should not be distributed . . . except on a prescription basis." In any case, whether it was for this or other reasons, the penicillin dentifrices did not continue on the market. Apart from commercial considerations, this may have been a premature development because even if penicillin could not be used in everyday dentifrices, a penicillin dentifrice might have had some usefulness in short-term treatment of patients with otherwise uncontrollable dental decay. It is also possible that using antibiotics in other ways might be justified in physically handicapped or mentally deficient patients, where ordinary methods of caries control cannot be used.

The last phase of experimentation with antibiotics has been directed mainly towards investigating the role of infection with specific microorganisms in experimental caries. Following the finding that transmission of microorganisms was important in initiating active caries in animals, it became important to establish the specificity of the bacterial types involved. After it was found that the caries seemed to result from oral contamination with the streptococcus from the feces, Keyes (*18*) was able to demonstrate that penicillin and erythromycin which eliminated such streptococcal types from the mouth also prevented caries. To demonstrate the specificity of specific strains of organisms, test streptococci were made streptomycin-resistant so that they could be used as markers and identified in the presence of other streptococcal types (*8*). This made it possible to show that the marked types were transmitted from one animal to another (*6*) and to identify them as the infective agents which produce caries in otherwise caries-free animals.

This technique of developing streptomycin resistance in specific strains of streptococci was used by Krasse *et al.* (*20*) to study "infection" of human mouths with exogenous cariogenic streptococci. He demonstrated long-term survival of a human cariogenic streptococcus after implantation in mouths in which it was previously absent. Cariogenic hamster streptococci survived for shorter periods.

Another way in which the antibiotics have been used to indicate the cariogenicity of specific bacterial types is by using them as Guggenheim *et al.* (*10*) have done to depress the usual oral flora to produce a partial gnotobiosis so that the introduced test type will face a less competitive struggle for existence and become established in a situation in which it would not otherwise survive. Using a similar approach, Bowen (*1*) was able to show that an erythromycin-resistant streptococcus from human teeth could be established in the mouths of monkeys rendered partially gnotobiotic by administration of erythromycin.

A further use for antibiotics in caries research has been to indicate the importance of bacterial polysaccharides in the sticky masses or plaques which form on the tooth surfaces of rats and hamsters on a sucrose diet (*19*). Since tooth destruction occurs under these plaques, agents which will inhibit the streptococci responsible for their formation would have potential importance in the prevention of caries in man. Keyes (*19*) has shown that in rats and hamsters daily short applications of penicillin, erythromycin, streptomycin, tetracycline, and speramycin are very effective in preventing plaque formation and subjacent tooth decalcification. Vancomycin was somewhat less so, and neomycin, bacitracin, and thiostrepton without effect. While caution cannot be too strongly emphasized in projecting animal findings to conditions in man, Mitchell and Holmes (*30*) have demonstrated that frequent applications of vancomycin will prevent the development of one type of plaque deposit in human mouths.

In conclusion, a final question has to be faced—that is, whether repeated use in the mouth of a therapeutic vehicle containing a "safe" antibiotic free of all medical hazards would be wise. If it killed a wide spectrum of oral bacterial types, its use would not be without danger because elimination of the predominant bacterial types in the mouth might allow other organisms, such as fungi, to become established, with possible unfortunate pathological effects. The perfect anticaries antibiotic will need to have preferential antagonism for only those types which are particularly important in caries causation and no effect on other types. Achieving this goal should not be beyond the possibilities of future research.

### *Literature Cited*

(1) Bowen, W., personal communication, 1968.
(2) Brudevold, F., Bibby, B. G., unpublished findings.
(3) Brudevold, F., Hawes, R. R., *J. Dental Res.* **1952,** 31, 474.
(4) Falla, W. S., Shaw, J. H., *Arch. Oral Biol.* **1965,** 10, 537.
(5) Fitzgerald, R. J., Jordan, H. J., *J. Dental Res.* **1955,** 34, 685.
(6) Fitzgerald, R. J., Keyes, P. H., *Am. J. Pathol.* **1963,** 42, 7.
(7) Fitzgerald, R. J., Keyes, P. H., *J. Am. Dental Assoc.* **1960,** 61, 9.
(8) Fitzgerald, R. J., Zander, H. A., Jordan, H. J., *J. Am. Dental Assoc.* **1950,** 41, 62.
(9) Fosdick, L. S., Ludwick, W. E., *J. Dental Res.* **1950,** 29, 664.
(10) Guggenheim, B., Konig, K. G., Muhlemann, H. R., *Helv. Odont. Acta* **1965,** 9, 121.
(11) Handelman, S. L., Hawes, R. R., *Arch. Oral Biol.* **1965,** 10, 353.

(12) Handelman, S. L., Hawes, R. R., *J. Oral Therap. Pharmacol.* **1964,** 1, 23.
(13) Handelman, S. L., Mills, J. R., Hawes, R. R., *J. Oral Therap. Pharmacol.* **1966,** 2, 338.
(14) Hawes, R. R., Thesis, University of Rochester, Rochester, N. Y., 1951.
(15) Hill, T. J., Kniesner, A. H., *J. Dental Res.* **1948,** 27, 267.
(16) Hill, T. J., Sims, J., Newman, M., *J. Dental Res.* **1953,** 32, 448.
(17) *J. Am. Dental Assoc.* **1952,** 45, 466.
(18) Keyes, P. H., *Arch. Oral Biol.* **1960,** 1, 304.
(19) Keyes, P. H., *J. Oral Therap. Pharmacol.* **1966,** 3, 157.
(20) Krasse, B., Edwardsson, S., Svensson, I., Trell, L., *Arch. Oral Biol.* **1967,** 12, 231.
(21) Lind, H. E., *Antibiot. Chemotherapy* **1954,** 4, 161.
(22) Lind, H. E., Zander, H. A., *J. Dental Res.* **1950,** 29, 667.
(23) Law, F. E., Wallace, D. R., Spitz, G. S., *Public Health Rept.* **1961,** 76, 1094.
(24) Lewis, Charles N., M.D., personal communication, 1952.
(25) Littleton, N. W., White, C. L., *J. Am. Dental Assoc.* **1964,** 68, 520.
(26) Ludwick, W. E., Fosdick, L. S., Schantz, C. W., *J. Am. Dental Assoc.* **1951,** 43, 285.
(27) Mahler, I. R., Manly, R. S., *J. Am. Dental Assoc.* **1958,** 56, 854.
(28) McClure, F. J., Falk, J. E., Rust, J. D., *J. Am. Dental Assoc.* **1956,** 53, 1.
(29) McClure, F. J., Hewitt, W. L., *J. Dental Res.* **1946,** 25, 441.
(30) Mitchell, D. F., Holmes, L. A., *J. Periodont.* **1965,** 36, 202.
(31) Muhlemann, H. R., Meyer, R. W., Konig, K. G., Marthaler, T. M., *Helv. Odont. Acta* **1961,** 5, 18.
(32) Pindborg, J. J., *Acta Odont. Scand.* **1958,** 16, 383.
(33) Rosen, S., Ragheb, C. A., Hoppert, C. A., Hunt, H. R., *J. Dental Res.* **1956,** 35, 399.
(34) Shaw, J. H., Sweeney, E. A., *J. Dental Res.* **1957,** 36, 349.
(35) Shiere, F. R., *J. Dental Res.* **1957,** 36, 237.
(36) Stephan, R. M., Fitzgerald, R. J., McClure, F. J., Harris, M. R., Jordan, H. J., *J. Dental Res.* **1952,** 31, 421.
(37) Stephan, R. M., Harris, M. R., Fitzgerald, R. J., *J. Dental Res.* **1952,** 31, 475.
(38) Volker, J. F., Apperson, L. D., King, W. J., *J. Dental Res.* **1955,** 34, 733.
(39) Walsh, J. P., Smart, R. S., *New Zealand Dental J.* **1951,** 47, 118.
(40) Webman, H., Kniesner, A. H., Hill, T. J., *J. Dental Res.* **1948,** 27, 258.
(41) Welsh, H., Randall, W. A., Buckman, L. E., Hendrix, F. D., *Antibiot. Chemotherapy* **1952,** 2, 249.
(42) White, B. J., Kniesner, A. H., Hill, T. J., *J. Dental Res.* **1949,** 28, 267.
(43) Zander, H. A., *J. Am. Dental Assoc.* **1950,** 40, 569.
(44) Zander, H. A., Bibby, B. G., *J. Dental Res.* **1947,** 26, 365.
(45) Zander, H. A., Lisanti, V. F., Shiere, F. R., *J. Dental Res.* **1951,** 30, 139.

RECEIVED October 27, 1969.

# 6

# Other Organic Compounds and Dental Caries

KENNETH O. MADSEN

Dental Branch, University of Texas, Houston, Tex.

*Caries in experimental animals may be influenced by the dietary administration of a wide variety of organic compounds. Some influences are attributed to physiological or pharmacological effects. Phenolic acids, polyphenols, antioxidants, antienzymes, carbonyl binding agents, and complexing agents as well as organic polymers all affect caries production. Anticaries activity was widespread in the outer coverings of seeds under all conditions studied. Naturally occurring anticariogenicity was also noted in unrefined sugar products, cocoa, and chocolate.*

Many naturally occurring and synthetic organic substances when added to the diet have an influence on caries. Some, including organic phosphates and fluorides, have been reviewed elsewhere in this symposium. Primarily, the results from compounds that influence caries in experimental animals will be discussed in this paper. Most of the compounds tested in clinical studies as components of toothpaste, mouthwashes, and chewing gum have been reviewed in detail elsewhere (*48, 146, 149*) and will be considered here in summary manner.

Thousands of compounds have been screened by a variety of *in vitro* testing procedures, most involving microbiological assays where microorganisms came from saliva or dental plaque or are strains suspected of being important in the caries process. Usually, the effect of the compound on total acid production, pH, or growth is measured. Shaw concluded in 1959 in an excellent review of caries-inhibiting agents (*149*) that "no specific *in vitro* test procedure has been shown to have a sufficiently good correlation with clinical trials to merit confidence."

Such testing, of course, provides one means for finding suitable compounds for subsequent trial at the experimental animal stage prior to clinical evaluation. Although it is appropriate to mention the most likely compounds discovered in screening and *in vitro* tests, primarily only those compounds tested both *in vitro* and in experimental caries assays will be considered in this discussion.

The compounds considered will be classified arbitrarily on the basis of certain of their chemical similarities, on whether or not they appear to have a specific action on caries, and whether their effect on caries may be a consequence of their physiological or pharmacological activity.

The array of factors influencing each of the different dental caries studies cited in this review was not only large but often difficult to determine. Accordingly, the factors included in the description of each assay were those considered most significant either for the particular study or for comparing it with other studies. Whenever it appeared that a substance or compound had had a statistically significant or other valid effect on caries, such has been stated simply. No attempt has been made to describe the extent of the effects—*e.g.*, percentage inhibition—since this type of evaluation is highly relative and somewhat misleading. If effects can be established as real, or not, it is assumed that they can be made more or less dramatic by varying assay conditions. The assay conditions have been described in detail when effects were found.

### *Materials and Methods*

Although this paper is primarily a review, some pertinent new data from the author's laboratory will be discussed. These data were obtained by methods similar to those previously described (*109, 110, 112*).

In the early studies with or related to seed hull anticaries activity (*108, 110, 111;* Table I) and with cedar wood, cotton rats were placed on the cariogenic diet as 18-day-old weanlings for 14 weeks, after which caries scores for all three molars were measured and reported.

**Table I. Comparison of Caries and Decalcification Inhibiting Abilities of Diets Containing Seed Coverings**

| *Group* | *Material Studied* | *Caries Assay*[a] *No. Carious Lesions, Mean ± S.E.M.* | *In vitro Assay* | |
|---|---|---|---|---|
| | | | *Enamel Dissolved, Mg* | *Acid Produced, Ml, 0.05*N |
| 1 | None | 25.8 ± 1.2 | 1.7 | 26.4 |
| 2 | Rice hulls | 17.3 ± 2.2 | 1.1 | 20.7 |
| 3 | Cottonseed hulls | 20.5 ± 3.1 | 1.0 | 28.1 |
| 4 | Peanut hulls | 18.2 ± 3.7 | 0.6 | 23.8 |
| 5 | Pecan hulls | 16.7 ± 2.3 | 0.9 | 31.3 |
| 6 | Rice bran (solvent-extracted) | 19.0 ± 1.7 | 0.5 | 28.0 |

[a] Control score significantly reduced by all materials fed; $P < 0.001$ (*110*).

**Table II. Effects of Short and Long Term Feedings of Organic Phosphates on Caries Scores of Cotton Rats**

| *Group* | *Phosphate Fed* | *No. Rats* | *No. Carious Molars, Mean ± S.E.M.* | *Extent of Carious Lesions, Mean ± S.E.M.* |
|---|---|---|---|---|
| | | Experiment 1[a] | | |
| 1 | None | 8 | 16.5 ± 1.7 | 33.9 ± 3.9 |
| 2 | $Na_2HPO_4$ | 8 | 18.3 ± 0.7 | 37.4 ± 1.6 |
| 3 | $(NH_4)_2HPO_4$ | 6 | 16.3 ± 1.2 | 33.5 ± 2.8 |
| 4 | Sodium phytate | 6 | 19.3 ± 1.3 | 39.5 ± 2.9 |
| | | Experiment 2[b] | | |
| 1 | None | 12 | 9.3 ± 1.0 | 19.3 ± 2.9 |
| 2 | Fructose 1,6-Diphosphate | 10 | 9.5 ± 1.2 | 20.0 ± 2.8 |

[a] Scores of first and second molars at 40 days of age.
[b] Scores of first molars at 30 days of age.

**Table III. Effect of Graded Exposures to Dietary Pancreatin on Caries Production and Salivary Glands of Cotton Rats**

| | | | | | *Salivary Gland Wts., Mg*[a] | |
|---|---|---|---|---|---|---|
| *Group* | *Days Fed* | *No. Rats* | *No. Carious Molars*[a] | *Body Wt*[a] | *Actual Wt.* | *Per Gram of Body Wt.* |
| 1 | 0 | 8 | 18.4 ± 1.0 | 50.3 ± 4.4 | 205.5 ± 14.9 | 4.44 ± 0.35 |
| 2 | 3 | 6 | 15.1 ± 3.1 | 47.7 ± 8.0 | 221.6 ± 45.2 | 4.24 ± 0.23 |
| 3 | 8 | 7 | 13.2 ± 2.7[b] | 53.0 ± 5.5 | 198.7 ± 21.4 | 4.56 ± 0.55 |
| 4 | 28 | 6 | 11.7 ± 3.9[b] | 53.7 ± 7.2 | 201.8 ± 22.4 | 4.85 ± 0.56 |

[a] Mean ± S.E.M.
[b] Control score significantly reduced; $P < 0.001$.

In later studies, we began the feeding assays with 12-day-old weanlings (*112*), terminating them at 30, 40, 50, or more days of age. Because of the developmental status of the teeth (*109*), total caries scores were reported for first molars, first and second molars, and for all three molars at these ages. In this manner, we studied certain phosphates (Table II, Expt. 1), pancreatin (Table III), and tetrahydroxybenzoquinone. The total caries scores for first and second molars at 40 days of age were reported in all cases except in the study with tetrahydroxybenzoquinone, where the scores for all three molars at 54 days of age were given.

A short-term assay whereby the agent tested was fed only a few days beginning at 12 days of age has also proved valuable, the residual effect on caries being measured in first molars at 30, 40, or 50 days of age. This assay was used to study the effect of short term exposures to seed hulls (Table IV) and pancreatin (Table III). Removing sucrose

**Table IV. Effect of Feeding Various Seed Coverings for Two Days on Caries Scores Observed at 50 Days of Age**

| *Group* | *Material Fed, 25% level* | *No. Rats* | *No. Carious Molars, Mean ± S.E.M.* | *Extent of Carious Lesions, Mean ± S.E.M.* |
|---|---|---|---|---|
| 1 | None | 8 | 9.8 ± 1.5 | 20.5 ± 3.8 |
| 2 | Peanut | 8 | 5.8 ± 1.1[a] | 11.4 ± 2.4[a] |
| 3 | Pecan | 7 | 7.4 ± 1.6 | 14.7 ± 3.1[a] |
| 4 | Rice bran (solvent-extracted) | 8 | 7.3 ± 1.1 | 14.0 ± 3.4[a] |

[a] Control score significantly reduced; $P < 0.001$.

**Table V. Effect of Feeding Various Hulls for Three Days on Caries Scores Observed at 30 Days of Age**

| *Group* | *Hulls Fed, 24% Level* | *No. Rats* | *No. Carious Molars, Mean ± S.E.M.* | *Extent of Carious Lesions, Mean ± S.E.M.* |
|---|---|---|---|---|
| | | Experiment No. 1 | | |
| 1 | None | 7 | 5.3 ± 1.1 | 10.3 ± 2.2 |
| 2 | Pearl rice | 6 | 2.0 ± 0.7[a] | 3.8 ± 1.4[a] |
| 3 | Calrose rice | 7 | 2.6 ± 1.2[a] | 5.1 ± 2.3[a] |
| | | Experiment No. 2 | | |
| 1 | None | 6 | 8.2 ± 1.2 | 16.3 ± 2.3 |
| 2 | Texas rice | 7 | 4.1 ± 00.9[a] | 7.9 ± 1.8[a] |
| | | Experiment No. 3 | | |
| 1 | None | 7 | 7.0 ± 1.8 | 14.0 ± 3.6 |
| 2 | Peanut | 7 | 3.9 ± 1.0[a] | 7.6 ± 2.1[a] |
| 3 | Autoclaved peanut | 6 | 5.2 ± 1.2 | 10.7 ± 2.6 |

[a] Control score significantly reduced; $P < 0.001$.

from the basal diet during this early exposure enhanced the effects of agents such as fluoride and seed hulls fed at this time (*113*). Sucrose, of course, was removed from the control diet as well. This feeding technique was used to study the effects of seed hulls (Table V), of a 4% dietary level of fructose-1,6-diphosphate (Table II, Expt. 2), and of pine cones and a peanut hull fraction.

The composition of the basal Diet 875 (*25, 172*) used in all studies contained 50% ground oats, 32% whole milk powder, and 18% sucrose with 2% of 1:20 liver powder. A fat-soluble vitamin supplement was given weekly. Groats were replaced either by the finely ground seed hulls under test or by an equal amount of cellulose in the control diet. When sucrose was removed during short-term feeding of a test agent, additional cellulose or groats was added to replace it. The large variation in amount of ground oats or cellulose *per se* did not influence caries (*114, 148*).

At the end of all studies, fissure caries was measured by the method of Shaw *et al.* (*153*), mean scores and the standard error of the mean (S.E.M.) were determined, and the significance of differences was determined by chi-square analysis.

Table VI provides a summary of the compounds studied for their effect on dental caries. Italics indicate that one or more investigators reported caries to be decreased, although others may have found no effect. Caries increases are noted. Asterisks identify new data on cotton rats from the author's laboratory.

**Table VI. Sequential Listing of all Materials and Compounds Cited from Either Animal or Human Caries Studies**

*Anticaries Activity of Seed Hulls*

*Occurrence and Geographical Distribution*

*hulls of oats, rice* (3 varieties*), *peanuts**, *barley*, *cottonseed*, *pecans* (shells)*; *solvent-extracted rice bran**; straws of oats, rye, barley, wheat; woods of fir, redwood, *cedar**; cones of loblolly*, spruce*

*General Chemical Nature of Seed Hull Activity*

*ethanol*, *ether*, *mild aqueous base*, or *acetone extracts of oat hulls*

*Mode of Action of Seed Hull Factors*

peanut hull fraction*, *sodium** or *calcium phytate*, *phytin*, *sodium β-glycerol phosphate*, dibasic sodium* or ammonium phosphates*, fructose-1,6-diphosphate*

*Other Protective Agents*

*Unrefined Sugars*

*brown sugar*, *black treacle* (calcium phosphate), sugar beets, *shredded beets in water*

*Cocoa and Chocolate*

chocolate milk, drink [slight increases?], *dark and milk chocolate* [increased, decreased], *fresh* or *roasted cocoa beans* or *neutralized ash*, *water soluble* (tannins?) *and insoluble fractions of non-fat cocoa powder*, *commercial tannins*, *tannic acid*, *mimosa* or *quebracho extracts*

*Other Caries Compounds*

*Phenolic Acids and Polyphenols*

"acidic fraction of ether solubles" from oat hulls: ferulic*, *p*-hydroxybenzoic*, *syringic**, vanillic*, sinapic, *p*-hydroxyphenylpropionic, *p*-coumaric acids; *p*-hydroxyphenylpyruvic*, 3-methoxy-4-hydroxy mandelic*, *caffeic**, veratric*, anisic*, gallic, 3-piperonylacrylic, mandelic, kojic, homovanillic, ethylhydrocaffeic, *o*-coumaric, quinic acids; lupulon; eugenol; *eugenol palmitate;* protocatechuic aldehyde or *acid; vanillin aldehyde* or acid, D-catechin; hesperitin methyl chalcone; hesperidin; esculin; *coumarin; hesperitin; naringenin;* naringin; N-*pro-*

**Table VI. Continued**

*pyl gallate* [increased, decreased]; *nordihydoguiarietic acid;* morin; usnic acid; rutin; quercetin; *theobromine; caffeine; xanthine*

*Antioxidants*

*butylated hydroxyanisole* or *toluene, 1,2-dihydro-6-ethoxy-2,2,4-trimethylquinoline,* ascorbic or isoascorbic acids, ascorbic acid plus α-tocopherol, butylated hydroxytoluene plus citric acid, thioglycolic acid [increased], dithiothreitol*; hydrogen peroxide [increased, decreased] zinc or sodium perborates [increased]

*Antienzymes*

*penicillin, sodium-*N*-lauroyl sarcosinate* (SLS), *sodium dehydroacetate* [increased, decreased], SLS plus dicalcium phosphate, *SLS plus sodium monofluorophosphate and sodium metaphosphate, stannous fluoride plus calcium pyrophosphate, sodium dehydroacetate plus sodium oxalate, sodium oxalate, sodium iodoacetate, urea, urea plus dibasic ammonium phosphate, d,*1-glyceraldehyde

*Carbonyl-Binding Agents*

*sodium* or *potassium metabisulfites, carboxylmethoxylamine hemihydrochloride, dimedone, sodium bisulfite, sodium hydrosulfite, sodium sulfite,* sodium sulfate, sodium bisulfate

*Complexing Agents*

ethylenediaminetetraacetic acid (EDTA) [increased], *oxalate* [increased, decreased], *copper* or magnesium [increased] or *sodium chlorophyllin, copper sulfate,* zinc or nickel or manganese acetates [increased], zinc or nickel or manganese or copper EDTA complexes, ferric acetate plus tannic acid [decreased?], potassium thiocyanate [increased], sulfanilamide [increased], 8-hydroxyquinoline, o-*phenanthroline* [increased, decreased], neocuproine, tetrahydroxybenzoquinone [increased]*, *sodium azide,* thiouracil [increased]

*Organic Polymers or Films*

agar, celluflour, *high* or *low molecular weight polyvinyl acetates, natural chicle, Arochem, acid-neutralizing anion exchange resins* (*soft resins*), anion exchange resins in chloride form [increased], silicone oil [increased], *fats,* oils, hydrocarbons, *tetradecylamine*

*Enzymes*

*pancreatin**; pancreatic amylase; α-amylase; α-amylase inhibitor; "rhozymes"*: A-4, 41, H-39, HP-150, lipase B, Pectinol 10-M; *lysozyme; dextranases*

*Disinfectants*

*Zephiran,* Zephirol, Bradisol, *merfen,* surfen, nitrofurazone [decreased?], *chloramine-T, histane*

*Caries Factors with Physiological and Pharmacological Activity*

*semicarbazide hydrochloride,* β-aminopropionitrile, cyanoacetic acid, cyanoacetamide, propionitrile, β-dimethylaminopropionitrile, ethylenecyanohydrin, *acetonitrile, thyroxine,* propylthiouracil [increased], *pilocarpine, malic acid,* sour or plain or sweet ciders, tripelennamine citrate

**Table VI. Continued**

[increased], thenyldiamine, chlorothenepyramine, methimazole, mestranol [increased], norethynodrel [increased], ethynestradiol [increased], medroxyprogesterone [increased], progesterone, estradiol [increased], diethystilbestrol [increased], estradiolbenzoate [increased], norethandrolone [increased, decreased], cortisone, hydrocortisone acetate [increased], corticosterone [increased], Diamox [increased]

*General Discussion*
*betadine**

### *Anticaries Activity of Seed Hulls*

Ideally, a caries-preventive agent should have no other action unless that action is beneficial. A promising source of anticaries activity that appears to have no effect except on experimental dental caries has been found in the outer coverings of various seeds.

**Occurrence and Geographical Distribution.** Constant, Phillips, and Elvehjem found in 1952 (*25*) that cotton rats fed the ground whole grains of corn, wheat, and oats developed less caries than when fed the processed products, corn flakes, wheat flakes, and oatmeal. This led to the discovery of anticaries activity associated with oat hulls (*26*). The ground hulls were caries inhibitory when fed at both 10 and 25% levels, either in a semipurified diet containing 67% sugar or in natural Diet 875 containing 18% sugar (*172*).

The oat hull factors were active under a wide variety of caries assay situations. Madsen (*108*) showed that 25% of dietary hulls in a semipurified diet containing 67% sucrose was effective when fed to Harvard strain of caries-susceptible albino rats. Buttner and Muhler (*17*) demonstrated the activity of 5 and 10% oat hulls fed to Sprague-Dawley albino rats in a natural, cariogenic corn–whole milk powder diet containing no added sucrose. McClure (*118*) found that 15% of hulls inhibited caries in Sprague-Dawley rats fed a corn–whole milk powder diet containing 25% sucrose. In all of these studies, fissure (occlusal) caries was studied; however, McClure (*118*) also showed that smooth surface lesions produced by a ground dry bread diet containing 18% cerelose were reduced by either 8 or 15% of oat hulls.

At the Wisconsin laboratory, the general occurrence of anticaries activity in the outer coverings of seeds was noted (*108*). The hulls of rice, peanuts, barley, and cottonseed fed at the 25% level decreased cotton rat caries produced by the 18% sucrose Diet 875. Different seed hull samples were caries inhibitory when fed at the 15% level in Diet 875 to another colony of cotton rats in Texas (*110*). In this study, anticaries activity was found in the hulls of cottonseed, peanuts, pecans (shells), three different varieties of rice hulls, and in solvent-extracted rice bran. The rice hulls were also active at the 5% dietary level.

The seed hulls fed in these studies had the following origins: oats and barley came from the Northern Midwestern States, rice hulls from the Gulf Coast (Texas and Louisiana), pecan and peanut hulls from Central and Northern Texas, and cottonseed hulls and peanut hulls from several Southeastern States.

Recently, the protective effects of hulls were demonstrated in hamsters. An Italian group (*54*) observed caries reductions with rice chaff and husks (hulls, presumably).

Recently, two varieties of rice hulls from California have been found active in cotton rat assays (Table V, Expt. 1). These hulls were assayed at 24% in the diet fed to weanlings for only 3 days, from 12 to 14 days of age. The basal cariogenic Diet 875 fed to both control and experimental groups contained no sugar during these 3 days. Diet 875 containing sucrose was then fed to both groups for a cariogenic period totaling 18 days. This was a severe test since it demanded that an early short-term exposure to hull activity be manifested for a prolonged period thereafter. Texas rice hulls were also active in this test (Table V, Expt. 2).

Other seed coverings were tested in an even more severe short-term feeding trial. The samples active in long-term studies (Table I; Ref. *110*) were used. The hulls were fed only during 12–13 days of age, with sugar present in the cariogenic diet at this time. All these brief early exposures to hulls significantly protected the teeth during the subsequent 35 days of cariogenic feeding.

The long-term effectiveness of a short exposure to hulls added to the practical significance of hull factors as caries-preventive agents.

In earlier comparisons (*108, 110*), the various hulls, except for cottonseed hulls, appeared equal in their anticariogenic activity. Cottonseed hulls from North Carolina and Alabama both were less active than other hulls. A high fluoride level reported for cottonseed hulls (*121*) argued against a synergism between hull factors and fluoride.

Negative results were obtained in caries assays of other woody plant materials fed at the 25% level to Harvard caries-susceptible rats (*108*). The straws of barley, rye, wheat, and oats were not caries inhibitory nor were the woods of Douglas fir, redwood, or incense cedar. More recently, Texas loblolly pine cones and Wisconsin spruce cones were assayed at the 24% level by the severe three-day assay used in Experiment 1, and no activity was found. On the other hand, 15% cedar wood fed to cotton rats for a 98-day cariogenic period inhibited caries. Mean incidence scores for all three molars for control and experimental groups were 23.1 and 17.6, respectively, $p < 0.001$ (*114*).

**General Chemical Nature of Seed Hull Activity.** The possibility that seed hull activity was caused by contamination by insecticide or fungi or by trace element composition seemed remote since activity was found in hulls from a wide geographical distribution. A significant role for fluoride was discounted (*17*).

Taketa and Phillips found that anticaries activity could be extracted from oat hulls with hot ethanol, ether, or mild aqueous base (*172*). The active extract contained the phenolic acids *p*-hydroxybenzoic acid, ferulic acid, and vanillic acid, as well as palmitic acid. Vogel, Thompson, and Phillips (*174*) continued this work and found the activity soluble in acetone, also. For their isolation work, they used hot ethanol extraction followed by ether and 5% sodium bicarbonate. To free the "acidic fraction of the ether solubles" containing phenolic acids and polyphenols from lipid, a pentane wash and acetone extraction were used. The data indicated that polyphenols rather than phenolic acids were the active agents. They characterized three flavanoids in the active extract, but to date none of these have been tested in a rat assay. The lability of the factors was suggested by the fact that none of their extracts or fractions was as effective in reducing caries as ground oat hulls *per se*. However, Taketa (*172*) showed that ethanol did not extract all the hull activity.

The lability of seed hull factors was also shown by the fact that the anticaries activity of rice hulls (*110*) and peanut hulls (Table V, Expt. 3) was at least partially destroyed by autoclaving. Recently, we found that peanut hulls, after grinding, lose activity during prolonged storage at moderate room temperature and that ground samples from commercial sources were inactive.

**Mode of Action of Seed Hull Factors.** Several observations have indicated that the hull factors may inhibit caries by their antibacterial activities. Taketa (*172*) found that about 5% of oat hulls was soluble in ethanol, and these solids inhibited caries as well as the growth of microorganisms from the carious lesions of cotton rats. *Lactobacillus acidophilus* acid production also was inhibited. Antibacterial activity was present in the acidic fraction of the ethanol extract. Similarly, this fraction from other seed hulls and from straws, pine cones, and a variety of woods inhibited acid production of *L. acidophilus* (*108*).

Madsen (*108*) confirmed the activity of the acidic fraction of the ethanolic oat hull extract. *L. acidophilus* was also inhibited by this same fraction prepared from the hulls of rice, peanuts, barley, and cottonseed as well as from straws, pine cones, and a variety of woods.

In another laboratory, Smales (*155*) noted the antibacterial effect of ethanolic extracts of oat hulls and wheat bran. Jenkins and Smales (*69*) confirmed this observation. They also found the aqueous extract of pecan hulls inhibited *Streptococcus lactis*, although peanut hulls exhibited only slight water-soluble activity.

Antibacterial activity may not always correlate with caries activity, however. The straws, cones, and some of the woods referred to above as having antibacterial activity were not anticariogenic (*108*). This was further illustrated by Eigen *et al.* (*32*) in a caries assay of a fraction prepared from peanut hulls. They used a glucose–saliva fermentation test and a cariogenic streptococcus species to guide the fractionation process and obtained most of the activity, as did Taketa, in a fraction containing phenolic acids. We tested their fraction at a level equivalent to 24% of dietary peanut hulls in the three-day test described in Experiment 3 (Table V), and found no activity. This was, of course, a severe test; yet with this test we repeatedly have found the crude peanut hulls to be active. This particular fraction had been stored under ordinary conditions for about 2 years. The possible lability of hull factors has been discussed and may be involved here.

The lack of specificity of the microbiological assays does not eliminate the possibility that hull activity is antibacterial or antienzyme. A depression of the cariogenic oral flora is the most ready explanation for the fact that early three-day exposures to the various hulls protected against caries for a subsequent 18 or 38 days of cariogenic diet (Tables IV and V). Earlier, we found that rice hulls fed only 10 days, from 18 to 28 days of age, were nearly as effective as when fed during the entire 98-day cariogenic period (*111*).

Seed hull factors may exert some of their effect by inhibiting tooth decalcification. Bibby, using the *in vitro* decalcification test of Andlaw (*2*), compared the ability of 15% hulls in Diet 875 to inhibit the enamel decalcification produced by Diet 875 alone. This test of our cotton rat diets showed that all the hulls inhibited decalcification, although the titratable acidity did not correlate with the decalcification values (Table I). As will be discussed later, this lack of correlation between the two tests has been a common finding in the *in vitro* assay of foods, and Bibby (*9*) believes that decalcification values may be the more meaningful criterion.

From a continuation of *in vitro* search for anticaries activity, Clarkson and Bibby (*24*) recently reported on a survey of 21 spices. Aqueous and alcoholic extracts inhibited both acid production and enamel decalcification in either bacteria–cereal or bacteria–glucose fermentation mixtures containing a cariogenic *Streptococcus salivarius*. Water-soluble ash factors and water- and alcohol-soluble organic factors were active in these tests. Some organic factors appeared labile, and compounds in addition to essential spice oils were probably responsible. Again, acid production did not correlate always with decalcification values.

Jenkins (*69*) showed the presence of decalcification inhibitors in the aqueous extracts of oat, peanut, and pecan hulls.

Phosphates will be discussed in detail in this symposium, but the suggestions by Jenkins (*70*) and more recently by Grenby (*53*) that seed hull activity is caused by organic phosphates should be mentioned, although they are based on *in vitro* data which may not predict the effect on caries satisfactorily.

McClure (*120*) found that sodium phytate inhibited smooth surface caries in Sprague-Dawley rats at 1.4 to 3.1% levels fed variously as phytin or calcium and sodium phytates. He noted that the total phosphorus of oat hulls did not correlate with their anticaries activity but suggested a role for organic phosphate of hulls (*118*). McClure found 4.5% sodium β-glycerol phosphate caries-inhibitory also (*122*), and similar data have been reported for the effectiveness of dietary phytate and β-glycerol phosphate against occlusal caries in white rats (*141*).

It seemed unlikely that the hull activity resulted from phosphates since we found that dietary supplements of inorganic or organic phosphates did not influence cotton rat fissure caries produced by Diet 875. Dibasic sodium and ammonium phosphates and sodium phytate fed in powdered form at the 2% level for a 28-day experimental period did not reduce caries (Table II, Expt. 1). In a short-term assay, fructose-1,6-diphosphate fed 3 days during 12–14 days of age also did not affect caries (Table II, Expt. 2).

Other investigators studied similar dietary levels of organic phosphates and reported negative findings. Limbasuta (*97*) found sodium phytate ineffective in the albino rat diet. Other workers found that sodium phytate did not influence hamster caries (*84*), nor did glycerol phosphate affect caries in rats (*93*). Under certain conditions, phosphates, especially organic phosphates, may not exhibit the anticaries activity generally found when inorganic phosphate salts were fed to rodents (*134*).

In summary, seed hulls appear to vary from one species to another and even between varieties of the same species with respect to the solubility and stability of their bacterial or decalcification inhibitors; these inhibitors, however, may not assure an anticaries effect. Quantitative differences in all of these activities are apparent. Finally, while systemic or pharmacological modes of action seem less likely than direct oral effects, they have not been eliminated as possibilities.

### *Other Natural Protective Agents*

**Unrefined Foods (Cereals).** A number of observations reviewed recently by Andlaw, Bibby, and Buonocore (*3*) have suggested that the anticaries activity present in unrefined cereals and in raw sugar products may protect the tooth against enamel decalcification. Osborn *et al.* (*137*) first postulated the importance of these protective factors and suggested organic phosphates as active agents. Subsequently, Jenkins (*70*) concluded that organic phosphates were the main factors that prevented enamel dissolution when unrefined flours, crude cane juice, and molasses were incubated with saliva, and that sodium phytate as well as unknown agents rendered these less refined products protective.

Recently, Grenby (*51*) showed that in both saliva and acid buffers whole wheat exhibited less decalcification than refined wheat. This activity was not destroyed by baking since both flours and breads were active; however, the activity was labile to phytase so that phytin (phosphorus) was implicated as an active component, as suggested earlier by Jenkins (*70*). Grenby (*52*) found the decalcification inhibitory activity in wheat bran but not in the germ fraction. He localized it in the aleurone layer, but not in the testa or pericarp.

Jenkins (*68*) presented further reasons for believing that phytate is involved in decalcification inhibition and stated that the otherwise chelating or decalcifying property expected from phytate was inhibited by an as yet unidentified cationic substance. His data showed that the decalcification inhibitors in brown bread and flour were water soluble and that the extracts decreased enamel solubility in acidic buffers alone. This indicated the inhibitors were protecting the tooth against acid rather than inhibiting the source of acid, namely, the salivary bacteria.

The inhibition of tooth substance decalcification by food–saliva mixtures has been studied. By various techniques, Andlaw (*2*) studied 28 foods, Soni and Bibby studied 30 foods (*156*), and Gillings (*46*) reported a study of 60 foods. Recently, Bibby and Weiss (*10*) reported decalcification and acid production values from *in vitro* incubation studies with *Streptococcus salivarius* for 90 wheat flours of different variety and geographical origin. The six-fold variation in decalcification values suggested a wide variation in the composition of the flours in this respect and perhaps in their effects on caries.

Some of the above studies and numerous similar reports were reviewed recently by Bibby (*9*). There was a disappointing lack of correlation between *in vitro* tests and the cariogenicities of foods as now known. There was also poor correlation between *in vitro* tests *per se*, so that foods could not be ranked according to their effects on acid production or decalcification. Moreover, where tested, most studies showed lack of correlation between pH, titratable acidity, and decalcification values. In general, less-refined foods, especially cereal products, caused less decalcification of tooth substance than did refined foods, even when the refined foods caused greater acidities.

Bibby's group believes that the inhibition of decalcification results primarily from inorganic factors since the ashes of several foods were active in decalcification tests (*2, 135*). However, organic factors were implicated in their study of spice extracts (*24*).

**Unrefined Sugars.** There has been a renewal of interest in comparing crude and refined sugars. Jenkins (*68*) confirmed that raw cane juices and molasses (black treacle) caused less decalcification *in vitro* than more refined sugar products such as brown sugar, honey, and a syrup. His data indicated that some of the activity arose from calcium although the greater portion of the activity was unidentified.

It remained for Stralfors (*163*) to establish that the factors in unrefined sugars were anticariogenic. He showed that hamster caries was decreased by dietary brown sugar whether it was fed at 50% in the diet as a dry powder or at 40% in drinking water. The activity was heat stable since a 35% level of the brown sugar baked into bread was protective. Twenty per cent of black treacle in the drinking water also was active against caries.

Like Jenkins (*68*), Stralfors found the protection was enhanced by calcium. However, in this case, dibasic calcium phosphate was used, and in light of current knowledge of phosphate anticaries activities in rodents (*134*), it was probably the phosphate (0.33% added phosphorus) rather than the calcium that was responsible.

Stralfors further observed that sugar beets *per se* were not inhibitory, but a mixture of shredded beets in water had anticaries activity. He postulated that polyphenol oxidases may act to produce the active substances, perhaps melanins, in the beet suspension, whereas melanoidins formed in Maillard reactions may be the active agents formed during raw sugar processing as in the production of treacle. With regard to the activity of brown sugar against hamster caries but not against decalcification in Jenkins' test (*68*), it was possible that the latter used cane sugar rather than the beet sugar used by Stralfors. Future studies should distinguish between the two sources.

A further consideration was raised by Konig and Muhlemann (*92*), who tested the same brown sugar studied by Stralfors, howbeit in Osborne-Mendel rats. They attributed the anticariogenicity of brown sugar entirely to the cleansing action of its coarse particles.

**Cocoa and Chocolate.** In his classical "Vipeholm Studies," Gustafsson *et al.* (*56*) noted that the caries produced in a group of patients eating chocolate was less than expected. Supplements of chocolate in milk and in a chocolate drink had no significant effect on caries in Harvard caries-susceptible rats, although increased caries could have been expected because of the sugar content of chocolate (*152*). Similarly, Dunning and Hodge (*31*) recently reported nonsignificant increases in caries in an institutional study of patients given 1 pint of chocolate milk per day and a slight benefit of milk containing cocoa and artificial sweetener. In marked contrast to these findings, Ishi, Konig, and Muhlemann (*64*) reported that milk chocolate and chocolate wafers produced more fissure and smooth surface caries in Osborne-Mendel rats than did 5 other between-meal snack foods in which orally fermentable and retentive carbohydrates, including sucrose, were present.

Recently, Stralfors (*165*) fed 20% chocolate in a hamster diet. Dark chocolate with 4% cacao mass inhibited caries more than did milk chocolate with 0.8% cacao mass. The presence of chocolate ingredients other than cacaos mass and the processing involved in chocolate manufacture did not alter the response from that observed in his prior experiments where cocoa powder, *per se*, was fed as described below.

Rozeik *et al.* (*140*) noted that 25% of dietary cocoa beans, either fresh or roasted, inhibited caries in sialoadenectomized albino rats, and he attributed most of the activity to the ash fraction. Kinkel and Newiger (*86*) found that 2% of cocoa ash only slowed the initiation of caries but that neutralized ash maintained a low caries score in rats. Later experiments comparing cocoa ash with mixtures of reagent salts (*85*) gave anticaries results that could be interpreted as caused by phosphates in both materials since phosphates are so active against rodent caries (*134*).

The early interests in cocoa were resumed by Stralfors (*160*), who observed that whole cocoa powder inhibited hamster caries by 84, 75, 60, and 42% when fed at 20, 10, 5, and 2%, respectively, in a natural basal diet containing 50% sugar. He noted that the activity was in the nonfat portion of the cocoa. Further study (*161*) showed that the nonfat powder contained both water-soluble and nonwater-soluble cariostatic fractions.

A detailed review of Stralfors' subsequent work is appropriate since it now appears that cocoa and chocolate activity acting against hamster caries includes organic compounds and that these may be related to many compounds described in this review.

In a further study of the water-soluble anticaries factors in cocoa, Stralfors (*162*) utilized a 1:15 water extract of defatted cocoa powder containing 1.5% of solids. This extract dried onto the potato starch portion of the diet inhibited hamster caries by 50%. The active fraction comprised half the weight of extracted solids, and it absorbed completely on activated charcoal. About 25% of the solids contained about half the anticaries activity and was nondialyzable and ash-free. By indirect evidence, it appeared to consist of tannins. The high and low molecular fractions appeared almost entirely organic but remained unidentified; however, Stralfors (*164*) later reinforced the probability that tannins may be important by showing that commercial tannins were also anticariogenic in his hamster assays. Hydrolyzable tannic acid was active at only 0.01% of the diet, while the condensed tannins in mimosa and quebracho extracts were active at 0.05 and 0.2%, respectively.

**Nature of Anticaries Activity of Cocoa and Chocolate.** In contrast to the seed hull factors already described, the cocoa factors did not appear alcohol-soluble, although there was a nonwater-soluble fraction present. Stralfors (*164*) believes that tannins and theobromine, which comprise at least 14 and 3.5%, respectively, of fat-free cacao mass (*20*), are the most likely water-soluble factors contributing to the anticariogenicity of cocoa. It appeared unlikely that inorganic (ash) factors, including phosphate and fluoride, were the anticaries factors because the extracts had a low ash content; charcoal absorption removed the anticaries activity but did not lower the ash value.

On the other hand, if the cacao factors are organic, their stability through the many procedures involved in cocoa and chocolate manufacture is noteworthy. The conching process of chocolate manufacture involves Maillard reactions as well as further oxidation of cacao tannins and loss of some volatile compounds from the cacao mass (*78*). The stability of the cacao factors was in contrast to the unstable nature of the seed hull factors in many instances. Although both activities appeared related to polyphenols—using the classification by Bate-Smith (*8*)—flavanones and hydroxycinnamic acids may be involved in seed hulls, while tannins and leucoanthocyanins may be involved in cacao bean products.

The cacao factors could act as antibacterial agents since cocoa and chocolate inhibit staphylococci in pastry fillings (*18*). Fuller *et al.* (*42*) noted that these materials inhibit some bacterial growth in milk and suggested that tannins were the responsible agents. Theobromine is also toxic to some bacteria (*138*). Unheated or autoclaved 5% concentrations of cocoa inhibit the growth of salmonella species (*16*). Both anaerobic and aerobic cultures of saliva were strongly inhibited by 5 and 10% concentrations of cocoa in the medium (*7*).

On the other hand, Jenkins (*69*) showed a potent decalcification-inhibitory activity for cocoa. Moreover, Stralfors (*160*) discounted the probability that chocolate would inhibit salivary acid production.

The possibility that caffeine and other similar compounds in the cocoa decreased caries by stimulating salivary flow became less likely by the fortunate use by Rozeik *et al.* (*140*) of albino rats whose salivary glands had been removed.

### *Other Caries Compounds*

For many caries-active compounds, their mode of action on caries production has been postulated on the basis of chemical or microbiological activities and whether or not they have effects in the body other than on caries. All the following compounds and categories of compounds are not without effect on over-all health, as exhibited by effects on weight gain, for example. However, they represent activities that conceivably could be employed in some caries-preventive procedure.

**Phenolic Acids and Polyphenols.** The strong evidence that seed hull anticaries activity was caused by certain phenolic acids and polyphenols led to testing a number of these compounds in caries assays. The widespread occurrence of such compounds in foods and their apparently general lack of toxicity enhanced their practical value as potentially useful dietary additives. Unique compounds may be expected in seed hulls since seed coats often contain organic constituents not found in the rest of the plant (*8*).

Vogel (*174*) identified the following phenolic acids in his active extracts (the "acidic fraction of the ether solubles") of oat hulls, and found them inactive in a cotton rat assay when included in a semipurified diet containing 67% sucrose: ferulic, *p*-hydroxybenzoic, syringic, vanillic, sinapic, *p*-hydroxyphenylpropionic, and *p*-coumaric acids. We have assayed all but the last three of these compounds in the cotton rat at the 0.1% level in natural Diet 875 containing 18% sucrose and have found no activity (*114*). We also found no activity for *p*-hydroxyphenylpyruvic acid, 3-methoxy-4-hydroxymandelic acid, caffeic acid, veratric acid, and anisic acid when tested similarly (*114*).

Later, Thompson, Vogel, and Phillips (*173*), summarizing 6 years' work by the Wisconsin group, verified the inactivity of sinapic, *p*-coumaric, and ferulic acids, and also noted the inactivity of gallic and caffeic acids, 3-piperonylacrylic acid, mandelic acid, lupulon, kojic acid, and eugenol. Muhlemann *et al.* (*128*) reported negative results for vanillic and homovanillic acids fed at the 0.2% level to albino rats. Jordan *et al.* (*72*) reported no effect for the ether ester of 3,4-dihydroxyphenylpropionic acid (ethyl hydrocaffeate). The results from many assays appeared to support the earlier conclusion by Vogel *et al.* (*174*) that phenolic acids were not, in general at least, the most active agents contained in the oat hull extracts nor perhaps in other hull extracts. Nevertheless, the Wisconsin group obtained significant caries reduction with syringic acid and eugenol palmitate, even though eugenol *per se* was ineffective (*173*). In their earlier report, palmitic acid alone was without effect (*174*). Apparently no other attempt was made to study synergistic effects between phenolic compounds and fatty acids.

Recently, Stralfors (*166*) fed 0.2% of phenolic compounds and confirmed the inactivity of ferulic, *p*-coumaric, and gallic acids and showed, also, *o*-coumaric and quinic acids to be inactive in a 50% sucrose, natural diet fed to hamsters. Protocatechuic aldehyde was inactive also; however, protocatechuic acid and caffeic acid were significantly anticariogenic in these studies. Under the same assay conditions the aldehyde of vanillin inhibited hamster caries (*164*). Smooth surface caries was inhibited more than fissure caries. Vogel (*174*) and Muhlemann *et al.* (*128*) found vanillic acid inactive in cotton and white rats, respectively.

The Wisconsin group (*173*) also reported the effects of a number of polyphenols of which D-catechin, hesperitin methyl chalcone, and hesperidin were all significantly anticariogenic at 0.2–0.3% in the semi-purified diet of cotton rats. Catechin was inactive, however, in the hamster assay of Stralfors (*166*), as was the coumarin, esculin. Coumarin, *per se,* decreased hamster caries but also depressed growth severely.

The effect of hesperidin in cotton rats was greater than that of its aglycone, hesperetin. Hesperidin increased caries significantly at the 0.5% level in Sprague-Dawley rats (*72*). These data did not confirm the work of Gustafsson and Krasse (*55*), who noted that antibacterial effects were restricted to the aglycones of flavanones. They reported that the aglycone naringenin was caries-inhibitory at the 0.1% level in the hamster diet. The Wisconsin group found no effect in cotton rats at the 1% level. No effect was found in Osborne-Mendel rats with 0.2% naringenin. Stralfors found the glycosides, naringin and hesperidin, to be inactive at 0.2% in hamster caries assays (*166*).

Further inconsistencies among assays of various workers were noted in testing the antioxidant polyphenol *N*-propyl gallate. This compound significantly enhanced cotton rat caries (*173*), yet decreased caries in Sprague-Dawley rats (*72*) and in hamsters (*98*). This discrepancy could not be related to slight differences in the weight gains of the animals fed *N*-propyl gallate in the three studies.

Another antioxidant polyphenol, nordihydroguaiaretic acid, studied in the same investigations, did not influence cotton rat or albino rat caries but reduced hamster caries when provided at 0.01% in drinking water. In another hamster study, 0.2% of this compound in the diet also decreased caries; however, growth was depressed (*166*).

The Wisconsin workers (*173*) found morin, usnic acid, and rutin inactive. Rutin also was inactive in albino rats (*72*). Rutin and morin were inactive in the hamster; however, another flavanol, quercetin, reduced hamster caries significantly when fed at 0.2% level in a 50% sucrose, natural diet (*166*).

Unfortunately, the three polyphenols identified from the active extract of oat hulls by Vogel and Phillips (*174*) have not been assayed. These were the flavanoids tricin (3′,5′-dimethoxy-4′,5,7-trihydroxyflavone), homoeriodictyol (3′-methoxy-4′,5,7-trihydroxyflavanone), and the chalcone corresponding to homoeriodictyol. The flavone, tricin, occurs very commonly in the Gramineae family (*8*), and the general bacteriostatic action of the flavanoid class of compounds has been noted (*142*).

A careful survey of compounds present in the outer coats of seeds and a diligent testing of those substances would be far more profitable than the further arbitrary testing of related compounds from the laboratory shelf. On the other hand, Bate-Smith (*8*) has compiled enough data to show that this approach would be complex. More consistent results could be expected among investigators testing natural compounds, however, because of the general effectiveness shown for dietary oat hulls tested by a variety of assays.

The above contentions were reinforced by the recent report from Stralfors (*164*), who continued his search for cocoa factors and discovered further sources of anticariogenicity. He found that hamster caries was inhibited by 0.2% dietary theobromine and caffeine which are cocoa components. Although these agents inhibited growth, the parent compound, xanthine, was cariostatic at this level without depressing growth.

**Antioxidants.** As noted, the effects of antioxidants in the cotton rat diet were studied by the Wisconsin workers as a result of observed similarities to the oat hull anticaries factors. Cocoa beans are rich in unidentified antioxidants (*78*). Like oat hull factors (*172*), they are absorbed on charcoal and may be phenolic in nature. In contrast to the hull factors, they are mostly water soluble.

Jordan and co-workers have studied antioxidants in Sprague-Dawley rats because of a general interest in their effect on the caries process (*72, 73*). Lisanti and Eichel (*98*) were interested in the possibility that the anticaries effect frequently observed with dietary fat was caused by its content of antioxidants.

Some comparative data among the three groups of investigators has already been discussed. Butylated hydroxyanisole also was studied by these workers. It decreased caries significantly in cotton rats at the 0.5% dietary level (*173*) and in hamsters at the 0.01% level (*98*), while 0.05% did not influence caries in Sprague-Dawley rats (*72*).

Similarly, butylated hydroxytoluene decreased cotton rat caries but did not influence Sprague-Dawley rats. This compound was toxic at 0.5% in the diet in both species. Sprague-Dawley rats had significantly less caries when 1,2-dihydro-6-ethoxy-2,2,4-trimethylquinoline was fed, but this compound also was toxic at the 0.5% level. No anticaries effect was found in Sprague-Dawley rats fed ascorbic acid, isoascorbic acid, $\alpha$-tocopherol plus ascorbic acid, or butylated hydroxytoluene plus citric acid (*72*). We found that 5% dietary ascorbic acid had no effect on cotton rat caries (*114*).

Only four of 13 antioxidants studied by Jordan *et al.* (*72*) were antibacterial against a variety of bacteria, but two of these, *N*-propyl gallate and 1,2-dihydro-6-ethoxy-2,2,4-trimethylquinoline, were caries inhibitory. These workers concluded that antibacterial activity rather than antioxidant activity in general was the most important role of the agents studied. They cautioned, however, that the low solubility of most of the antioxidants tested made it difficult to compare their antibacterial and anticaries activities.

The studies with antioxidants in three different diets and three different species involve so many variables that it is impossible to cite those primarily responsible for the different responses found. Because of the natural occurrence of organic antioxidants and their increasing use in foods, their effect on caries merits more study since at present their role is obscured by meager and conflicting data.

Green (*50*) suggested that a high oxidation–reduction potential of saliva was associated with rampant caries. The ability of ethylenediamine tetraacetic acid, a cariogenic chelator, to maintain a metal at a high oxidation potential may be pertinent (*116*). Another cariogenic chelator, thioglycolic acid, is also a reducing agent. On the other hand, the potent reducing agent, dithiothreitol, had no effect on cotton rat caries when fed at 1000 ppm for 3 days followed by 100 ppm for a subsequent 25 days. Mean caries incidence for control and experimental groups were 17.4 and 14.5, respectively, and the difference was insignificant (*114*).

The effect of hydrogen peroxide has been variable also. Hamsters were completely protected by 3% hydrogen peroxide in the drinking water, and there was no adverse effect on growth (*98*). In Holtzman rats, extensive caries-like lesions and severe growth depression were produced by 1 and 1.5% hydrogen peroxide in drinking water (*115*). Zinc peroxide and sodium perborate gave similar results. However, the lesions were produced when a noncariogenic diet was fed, and typical carious lesions were not produced.

**Antienzymes.** Fosdick (*39*) introduced the term "antienzyme" and suggested that caries would be prevented best by using enzyme inhibitors ideally supplied along with cariogenic food items. He has tested antienzymes almost exclusively in dentifrices and mouthwashes.

The ability of 38 compounds to inhibit a pH change in plaque material after its exposure to sucrose solution was tested by Fosdick (*39*). He assumed that retention of the compound on the tooth plaque was of primary importance, and first chose 10 compounds that showed satisfactory retention. Of these, three compounds, the antibiotic penicillin, the hexokinase inhibitor sodium-*N*-lauroyl sarcosinate, and the fungicide sodium dehydroacetate, were selected on the basis of the pH test. When selected subjects employed these in a mouthwash or dentifrice for a week, their plaque showed a decreased pH response to sucrose solution. Fosdick (*37*) also compared a dentifrice containing a detergent having no ability to bind to dental plaque with sodium-*N*-lauroyl sarcosinate (SLS) and after 2 years found about a 50% reduction in the caries experience of 1159 subjects. Later, Frasher and Hein (*41*) studied 365 Mexican subjects whose water supply contained 0.9 ppm of natural fluoride and reported nearly 50% reduction among those using SLS in a dentifrice.

Forscher and Hess (*36*) were unable to confirm either the *in vitro* or the clinical data showing SLS to be of value and concluded that pH measurements were not suitable for screening procedures. In another clinical test, Backer-Dirks (*4*) reported no beneficial effects among children who brushed with SLS for 20 months. Similarly, in a study where a stannous fluoride dentifrice was effective, SLS was ineffective (*177*). Conversely, Hayden (*60*) reported significant benefit among a similar number of children after 1 year.

Combinations of SLS with other agents also have been tested. Kyes *et al.* (*94*) found no reduction in caries for a SLS dentifrice. Finn and Jamison (*34*) reported that a dentifrice containing SLS, sodium monofluorophosphate, and sodium metaphosphate was more effective than one containing SLS and dicalcium phosphate. The role of SLS alone was not determined; however, they also reported the less active of the two SLS formulations to be as effective as one containing stannous fluoride and calcium pyrophosphate.

In animal tests with dietary SLS, a lack of caries protection was noted in Osborne-Mendel rats (*128*). With SLS in a high carbohydrate diet, however, Haldi *et al.* (*58*) found significant decreases in both sialoadenectomized and intact rats. Since the pH on the rat tooth surfaces was not affected, an antibacterial effect for SLS was postulated. Zipkin (*179*) reported that 0.5% of SLS decreased both smooth surface and occlusal caries. Later, however, Keyes (*82*) reexamined the data and reported that only the smooth surface caries produced by a corn starch–cerelose–skim milk powder diet was reduced. Using the same diet, Keyes and White (*83*) again reported a significant but slight reduction in smooth surface caries, but sulcal lesions were unaffected. They stated from personal communications that three other well-known workers in the experimental caries field revealed a further lack of any impressive effect with SLS in rats or hamsters.

In the 1 clinical trial reported (*168*), the use of a dentifrice containing 0.75% of sodium dehydroacetate decreased caries by about one-half over a two-year period. Since the dentifrice contained an equal quantity of sodium oxalate, an agent known to either enhance or decrease animal caries (*61*), this study did not assess the value of dehydroacetate *per se*.

Sodium dehydroacetate enhanced smooth surface caries in rats when administered by diet, drinking water, intubation, or injection (*180*).

Muhlemann *et al.* (*128*) found no effect for this compound provided at 0.02% in the drinking water of rats.

Nearly 4000 compounds have been screened by Cerul and coworkers (*19*) for their ability to inhibit glycolysis. These workers reasoned that the continual use of an oral antibacterial agent would be undesirable and, like Fosdick, devised a test whereby compounds were measured for their ability to inhibit glycolysis by salivary sediment. They selected 80 of the most promising chemicals and made further screening tests on the basis of their oral availability, discarding all compounds that were highly retained on the dietary constituents of the cariogenic diet. This procedure was opposite to that used by Fosdick (*39*), who sought compounds that were retained on casein. Seven compounds passed the second screening procedure and were tested in the diet. Thirty-three other satisfactory compounds were tested in caries assays by topical application after dissolving them in aqueous solutions containing glycerol or propylene glycol and made viscous with honey or methylcellulose. Only dietary sodium iodoacetate, a caries inhibitor, proved active in these caries assays employing Osborne-Mendel albino rats.

Earlier, using the salivary sediment screening procedure, Mahler and Manly (*115*) found neither penicillin nor dehydroacetic acid capable of inhibiting pH changes in salivary sediment, but they did select sodium-*N*-lauroyl sarcosinate. Fosdick (*39*) found all three compounds capable of inhibiting glycolysis in his *in vitro* tests. The generally disappointing results indicate that reliable criteria have not been discovered or employed for screening compounds for their anticariogenic activities.

Urea, which can enter dental plaque and render it alkaline (*157*), may also act as an antienzyme against the cariogenic microflora which apparently thrive in an acidic environment. Kessel (*79*) found the effectiveness of urea in reducing the oral *L. acidophilus* count was enhanced when dibasic ammonium phosphate (DAP) was used in various ratios along with urea in a dentifrice.

The results of clinical trials by 11 different investigators using urea-containing preparations have been reviewed (*149, 175*). Mostly, dentifrices of the urea–DAP type were used, and, in general, negative findings or only mild reductions were reported in this and other countries. Preparations containing the higher concentrations of urea and DAP were most effective. A urea–DAP dentifrice containing urease to enhance the release of ammonia was found ineffective (*59*). However, the use twice a day of a topical application of a 45% solution of urea alone decreased caries sharply in a small study (*159*).

The possibly greater effectiveness of fluoride-containing dentifrices has quieted, perhaps prematurely, the enthusiasm for testing some of the most promising organic compounds by adequate clinical procedures (*175*).

Topical applications of urea solutions or ammoniated dentifrices did not significantly influence caries in hamsters (*22, 81*) except at very high levels of application, where caries was increased. The inclusion of 1% dibasic ammonium phosphate and 0.6% of urea in the hamster diet caused major caries reductions (*22, 23*). In the light of the recent observations of anticaries effects of dietary phosphates, the hamsters may have responded to the provision of phosphate rather than to the basic reaction of the supplement. On the other hand, urea alone decreased caries in rats when it was included in the drinking water at 1000 ppm or at 2% in the diet (*119*). In another study, caries in Sprague-Dawley rats was decreased by 5% but not by 2.5% of dietary urea (*117*). *Streptococcus salivarius* isolated from the saliva after urea feeding had high ureolytic activity. Hein (*61*) compared the effects of urea in rodents and concluded that the rat was more sensitive than the hamster.

Fosdick and Calandra (*38*) used an enamel–saliva incubation test and found that D,L-glyceraldehyde decreased enamel decalcification. Shaw (*147*) found no anticariogenic activity in either cotton rats or albino rats at the 0.5, 1, or 2% dietary levels of this compound.

Sodium iodoacetate, a well-known enzyme inhibitor, has been found anticariogenic by all investigators. Hein (*61*) tabulated a comparison of effects in rats and hamsters receiving the compound by different modes of administration and at various levels. A dietary or water concentration of 20 ppm appeared to give a maximal anticaries effect in both the albino rat and hamster. In rats, a graded dosage of 2, 20, and 200 ppm gave a corresponding decrease in caries (*107*).

**Carbonyl-Binding Agents.** Another mode of altering the metabolic activity of cariogenic oral microflora was considered by Jordan and coworkers (*74*). Both sodium bisulfite and sodium metabisulfite reduced acid production in saliva (*29*), and Jordan *et al.* found that the growth of a large number of microorganisms was inhibited by metabisulfite *in vitro*. They found that at concentrations which did not inhibit growth, however, acid production was decreased. They reasoned that the usual glycolytic pathway of metabolism had been altered by the metabisulfite, which was capable of binding aldehyde and ketone intermediates important in glycolysis. This effect on yeast metabolism is well known (*133*). When these workers fed 0.15, 0.3, and 0.9% sodium metabisulfite to Sprague-Dawley rats, they found reductions in occlusal caries of 33, 64, and 77%, respectively (*74*). Neither rat growth nor food intake was affected by the compound. Another group of workers (*15*) found potassium metabisulfite inhibited rat caries, and curiously, noted depigmentation of the incisors in the protected animals.

Stimulated by this concept, Jordan *et al.* (*71*) compared carboxylmethoxylamine hemihydrochloride and sodium metabisulfite, which are binding agents for aldehydes and ketones, and dimedone, which binds only aldehydes, at dietary levels of 0.05, 0.3, and 0.4%, respectively. Striking reductions in caries were observed for all compounds. On the basis of their molar dietary concentrations, these compounds were effective against caries and a variety of microorganisms in the order cited. Carboxylmethoxylamine, the most effective, manifested toxicity, but the other compounds did not affect rat growth.

Jordan *et al.* found a variety of sulfites which inhibit caries (*73*). At a range of 0.35–0.57% (0.04 *M*) in the diet, sodium metabisulfite, sodium bisulfite, sodium hydrosulfite, and sodium sulfite reduced caries 74% or more without adverse effect on rat growth. Sodium sulfate and sodium bisulfate were inactive. Although all of the sulfites were antioxidants, they were also all germicidal, presumably because of formation of sulfurous acid in solution. These workers discounted the antioxidant role since they found earlier that antioxidants generally did not inhibit caries (*72*). They favored the carbonyl-binding role of these compounds.

**Complexing Agents.** The widespread influence of metal ions on metabolic events is well known, and the biological aspect of metal-binding by complexing, or chelating, agents has received widespread review and attention (*33, 143*).

The many factors seemingly operative in the carious process should respond to complexing agents. The fact that many miscellaneous compounds affecting caries now may be classified together under this heading seems to have been overlooked for the most part, and already there may be more information from this standpoint than has been considered hitherto.

Ethylenediamine tetraacetic acid (EDTA) has been well established as a cariogenic agent under certain conditions. EDTA increased the cariogenicity of a diet producing occlusal caries in rats (*178*). Stephan and Harris (*158*) have reviewed their earlier work, where they found that smooth surface lesions in rats were enhanced by dietary EDTA and that this effect was counteracted by increasing the level of dietary salt mixture. The fact that rats, made caries-inactive by dietary antibiotics, did not respond to EDTA indicated that EDTA operated to remove enamel anions provided by the carious attack but did not act alone to cause demineralization. On the other hand, the antibiotic treatment could have altered the cycylization of EDTA *via* coprophagy. In this regard, Larson *et al.* (*96*) have shown that intubated EDTA significantly increased caries while injected EDTA had much less effect. They cite the work of Forman *et al.* (*35*), which showed that intubated EDTA rapidly appeared in the feces and hence was available orally *via* coprophagy, while injected EDTA appeared mostly in the urine.

Hein (*61*) summarized the influence of oxalate, another chelator, on experimental caries. Caries was decreased markedly in the hamster, equivocally in the albino rat, and increased in the cotton rat. There has been no explanation for these differences. The high content of 0.72–1.18% oxalic acid in fat-free cacao mass (*125*) should be noted in view of the fact that Stralfors (*162*) found cacao anticariogenic in the hamster diet.

Several earlier studies on the chelates copper and magnesium chlorophyllin have been compared by Hein (*61*). Neither albino nor cotton rat caries was influenced significantly by the copper derivative, but hamster caries was dramatically reduced or increased by the copper or magnesium derivatives, respectively. Copper sulfate decreased hamster caries (*61*). This later observation was confirmed recently (*43*) when copper sulfate (but not a copper EDTA complex) was applied topically to hamster teeth. Chlorophyll-containing dentifrices were available for a time but have not been demonstrated of value. Recently, sodium chlorophyllin was found inactive against occlusal caries at the 0.2% level in the drinking water of Osborne-Mendel rats (*128*).

Hendershot and Forsaith (*62*) noted that the cariogenic effects produced by feeding zinc, nickel, and manganese as the acetates were removed by feeding these metals as EDTA chelates. These studies and those with chlorophyllins appear to be the only ones in which the effects of organic metal chelates on caries have been studied.

An *in situ* chelation of metal ions may be of benefit, as indicated by the traditional Japanese *Ohaguro* technique that stains teeth black and renders them somewhat caries and acid resistant (*65*). Alternate treatments with ferric acetate and tannic acid result in ferric tannate, which adheres to the teeth. A similar mechanism may be speculated for the anticaries effect reported from dietary tannins (*164*).

Another chelator, thiocyanate, is normally present in saliva (*28*). Sterile human parotid secretions contain antibacterial activity against *L. casei* (*28*), and Dogon *et al.* (*27*) reported the presence of two thiocyanate-dependent antibacterial systems where thiocyanate acts in conjunction with either peroxidase or another salivary protein.

Potassium thiocyanate was inactive against caries at 100 ppm in the drinking water of albino rats (*119*), while a trend for increased caries in the Osborne-Mendel rat was noted by Muhlemann and co-workers (*128*). In the latter study, two other chelators, *o*-phenanthroline and a sulfa drug, sulfanilamide, also tended to enhance caries, while the chelator 8-hydroxyquinoline was without effect. In another study with *t*-phenanthroline, weekly topical applications of aqueous solutions (1 mg/ml) to the teeth of Wistar white rats produced significant caries reductions (*76*).

In the same study, neocuproine was inactive. It appeared that both substances could bind to enamel and harden it.

The chelator tetrahydroxybenzoquinone is cariogenic in cotton rats when fed for 42 days in Diet 875 at the 0.5% level. Mean incidence scores for control and experimental groups were 20.6 and 28.7, respectively, $P < 0.001$ (*114*).

Thiocyanate and sodium azide, a chelator that eliminates hamster caries almost completely (*98*) at the 0.001*M* level in drinking water, both reduce blood pressure in man (*1*).

Thioglycolic acid (*119*), both a chelator and reducing agent, enhanced caries in albino rats drinking it at the level of 100 ppm in their water. It may be significant in light of the postulated salivary gland–thyroid relationship that the goiterogen thiouracil, which enhances caries, is a chelator (*132*).

As a class of compounds, the flavanoids, discussed in connection with anticaries factors in seed hulls, having chelating properties (*21*).

Chelators are associated with both increased and decreased caries experience in rodents. Albert (*1*) made the observation that biochemicals, contrasted to synthetic ones, are highly specific for metals and that metal-binding in cells, accomplished mainly by organic phosphates and members of the citric acid cycle, remains largely unexplored. McClure, however, recently used organic phosphate metabolic intermediates (*122*). Perhaps more attention should be given to the effect on caries of the more subtle and specific effects obtainable with biological metal-binding compounds.

**Organic Polymers of Films.** Another approach in the search for agents that affect caries concerns organic polymers and factors which influence them. Francis and Meckel (*40*) produced artificial "white spot" identical to early human enamel lesions when agar was provided in the saliva–glucose mixture bathing the enamel surface. Gray *et al.* (*49*) noted the necessity for agar, protein (gelatin), or salivary mucin for white spot formation.

These *in vitro* experiments may bear some relation to the study by Shaw (*148*) wherein nutritionally inert materials were studied, and the nature of the material produced significant differences in caries experience. Agar and celluflour had no effect, but 10% dietary supplements of both high and low molecular weight poly(vinyl acetate) caused significant decreases in caries, as did natural chicle and arochem (the esterification polymer of glycerol, fatty acid, and dimerized rosin). The teeth in the protected groups looked cleaner, and, in view of Francis' observation (*40*), the formation of a cariogenic film may have been prevented.

Anion exchange resins also affected caries production (*47, 151*). Twenty per cent of various anion exchange resins in the diet gave major caries reduction in Harvard caries-susceptible albino rats. The primary effect was attributed to their acid neutralizing ability since in the chloride form they did not inhibit caries (*151*). Particle size was relatively unimportant, but the softest resin was the most active, perhaps because it was retained to a greater extent on the tooth surfaces. Related possibly to the postulated role for polymers in the initiation of tooth films that promote caries was the fact that the chloride-saturated resins, having no exchange capacity, tended to increase caries.

Boyers *et al.* (*12*) studied the influence of another polymer, silicone oil. Daily topical applications had no effect, but 10 and 20% dietary levels enhanced caries in proportion to the amount fed. This agent possibly enhanced caries by increasing the oral retention of the diet, but a surface effect as postulated for fats could also be argued. High levels of dietary fat did not appear to increase retention, but did reduce caries (*67*).

Walsh and Green (*176*) studied the possibility of covering the enamel surface with an acid-resistant film and found that fats, oils, and hydrocarbons had little effect. In later studies, finding little effect with anionic and neutral agents, they turned to amines and found after testing a large number that tetradecylamine was one of the most active in ability to bind to the tooth surface and inhibit decalcification. This work was reviewed (*63*), and it was stated that dentifrice studies were underway. The report of one small clinical study (*106*) indicated a 44% reduction in caries by the group using a tetradecylamine dentifrice.

**Enzymes.** Another approach to caries inhibition is to affect food residues, organic films, and plaque on tooth surfaces by dietary enzymes. Sweeney and Shaw (*171*) observed that 1% dietary pancreatin (dried, defatted pancreas) significantly inhibited caries in Harvard albino rats. This activity was associated with a slight increase in salivary gland weight, however, and salivary gland function can affect caries production (*67*).

We determined that pancreatin (Nutritional Biochemicals Corp.) at the 1% level in Diet 875 decreased caries in cotton rats in a graded response to the length of time the substance was fed (Table III). There was no significant effect on the weights of the submandibular salivary glands either on an absolute or body weight basis, nor was there any effect on body weights.

It was unlikely that pancreatic amylase played a role in these pancreatin studies since a 0.5% level of this enzyme did not influence caries in diets containing ground wheat fractions (*90*). Likewise, neither 1% $\alpha$-amylase nor 0.001% of an amylase inhibitor influenced a low degree of cariogenicity produced by a cornstarch diet fed to Osborne-Mendel rats (*127*).

We also fed cotton rats a number of commercial, food-grade enzyme preparations (Rohm and Haas) at the 1% level in Diet 875, but with completely negative results at the end of 18 days (*114*). These enzymes included "Pectinol 10-M" (pectinolytic), "Rhozyme A-4" and "Rhozyme 41" (proteolytic with high and low diastase activity, respectively), "Lipase B" (lipolytic), and "Rhozyme HP-150" (hemicellulolytic).

In a similar assay, with a semipurified basal diet containing 43% of a cariogenic cornstarch at the expense of the sucrose portion of the diet, caries was not influenced by 1% "Rhozyme H-39" (diastatic). One per cent pancreatin was again highly protective (*114*). A correlation between a low caries incidence and a high salivary lysozyme level has been reported (*44*). One report indicated a caries-protective effect of dietary lysozyme (*30*), but other findings were negative (*126, 169*). Konig and Muhlemann (*91*) reinvestigated the effect with a level of 0.010% in two different diets and concluded that lysozyme had no appreciable influence on caries.

The negative results with dietary enzymes suggest that pancreatin may not be acting *via* its enzyme content. The fact that enzymes may be innocuous as dietary additives makes further testing attractive, however.

Recently, it has been discovered that microorganisms from the oral cavities of caries-active humans and animals elaborate a sticky, insoluble polyglycan (dextran) plaque especially from dietary sucrose as a substrate. Dextranases inhibit caries by preventing these plaques. A review of this fascinating area would entail scores of references; however, Gibbons (*45*) has reviewed many of the salient features. To maintain perspective, however, enzymes other than carbohydrases remain of interest since caries can be produced without sucrose and without dextran-containing plaques.

The antibacterial salivary peroxidase system in human saliva was mentioned earlier (*27, 28*). This system reportedly contains two major peroxidases (*66*) and two substrates, thiocyanates and hydrogen peroxide (*87*). Thiocyanate either was ineffective (*119*) or tended to increase caries (*128*), and hydrogen peroxide either decreased (*145*) or increased (*98*) caries. Peroxidase production by salivary glands may depend upon the nature of the oral microflora (*123*) and therefore on the nature of the diet. The effects of dietary salivary peroxidases have not been investigated. Indirect studies with peroxidase-containing and peroxidase-inactivated rice bran samples showed no correlation between peroxidase content and anticaries activities of the bran fed to cotton rats in Diet 875 (*114*). Nevertheless, it may be of value to make comparisons between peroxidase content of foods and their cariogenicities since this enzyme occurs widely in plant foods and is very stable (*13*). Lactoperoxidase and aspects of salivary peroxidase have been reviewed recently (*124*).

**Disinfectants.** Although many compounds have been used as disinfectants in mouthwashes, there is little evidence clinically or in animals that caries is significantly inhibited by them. In one small clinical study the frequent daily use of 0.1% Zephiran on the teeth resulted in less caries (*159*). Muhlemann *et al.* (*128*) recently reported negative results for several commercial disinfectants such as Zephirol, Bradisol, Merfen, and Surfen provided in the drinking water of rats, although 0.02% of dietary nitrofurazone may have significantly reduced occlusal caries in these animals. Stralfors (*167*) tested 1% of chloramine-T in the drinking water or in a 50% sucrose, natural diet for hamsters. By both modes of administration, caries was strongly inhibited.

In a later study in Muhlemann's laboratory (*139*), Merfen (phenyl mercuric borate) and Histane (chlorhexidine diacetate) were tested by brushing the teeth of Osborne-Mendel rats daily with 0.125–0.5% solutions in glycerol or water. All treatments significantly decreased both fissure and smooth surface caries. Glycerol did not alter treatment effectiveness. They postulated that binding to the plaque was more important than good diffusion properties in the selection of antibacterial–anticariogenic compounds.

### *Caries Factors with Physiological and Pharmacological Activity*

Many organic compounds affect caries production indirectly. It may be appropriate to consider them, as their wide variety of physiological and pharmacological activities illustrate the complexity of factors that may influence the caries experience of a given individual or the results of an animal experiment.

As a sequel to their interest in carbonyl-binding compounds, Jordan *et al.* (*75*) compared semicarbazide hydrochloride, a carbonyl binder producing osteolathyrism, with the lathyrogenic agent β-aminopropionitrile, which is not a carbonyl binder. Both of these compounds produced a decrease in occlusal caries in proportion to the level of compound fed. Since neither compound showed pronounced antibacterial effects, the authors suggested that their lathyrogenic activity influenced caries; the mechanism was not clear, however. Semicarbazide is, of course, a chelator.

The action of these compounds in a diet producing smooth surface lesions added complexity to the data since semicarbazide had no effect while β-aminopropionitrile increased the production of these lesions (*75*). Lathyrogens affect salivary gland morphology, however, (*77*) and the resultant effect on saliva might be expected to influence smooth surface caries more than occlusal caries.

Six nitriles related to β-aminopropionylnitrile but without lathyrogenic activity were tested for their ability to inhibit smooth surface caries. They were cyanoacetic acid, cyanoacetamide, propionitrile, β-dimethylaminopropionitrile, ethylene cyanohydrin, and acetonitrile. Only acetonitrile had a slightly inhibitory effect on smooth surface caries.

A review of earlier work (*144*) on the relationship of hormonal factors to caries indicated a high degree of interrelationship. Only passing mention will be made here of the more salient features and some recent observations.

Muhler *et al.* (*132*) summarized their work on the relation between the thyroid gland and the salivary glands of albino rats. Dietary thyroxine decreased dental caries while propylthiouracil, an antithyroid compound, enhanced caries. Thyroxine was associated with an increased salivary flow and a decreased salivary viscosity, whereas the opposite was true of propylthiouracil. These observations were consistent with the postulated importance of saliva as an oral clearance factor, as described by Jenkins (*67*) and shown by the pilocarpine experiment of Muhler *et al.* (*131*). Pilocarpine, a common sialogogue, caused increased salivation and decreased dental caries in white rats.

From the standpoint of providing an adequate salivary flow by normal physiological means, the use of saliva-stimulating tablets is noteworthy. Children sucking tablets containing malic acid, the major acid in apples, and sorbitol, a relatively nonfermentable carbohydrate (*150*), reportedly had decreased caries (*136*). However, no anticaries effect (*14*) was found in rats drinking an apple product. Sour, plain, or sweet ciders had no effect on caries. A decrease might have been expected because of the possibility for sialogogue action as well as the presence of tannins which have been shown anticariogenic by Stralfors (*164*).

Antihistamines frequently produce the complaint of xerostomia (dry mouth). There is one report (*130*) where antihistamines were provided as 12.5 and 50 mg % of tripelennamine citrate and thenyldiamine, respectively, in the drinking water of rats for 4 months. The former compound increased caries and the latter had no effect. In the diet at 0.1–0.2% neither of these compounds, nor chlorothenepyramine, influenced caries.

The observations of Haldi *et al.* (*57*) support those of Muhler *et al.* (*132*) that the thyroid–dental caries relationship is mediated by the salivary gland. Muhler *et al.* (*132*) compared the results of propylthiouracil treatment with that of two other goiterogens, potassium thiocyanate and methimazole. They found definitely less effect on caries, so the effect of goiterogens did not appear to be a general one which would always affect salivary glands and caries.

The relationship between caries and steroid hormones is complex and ill-defined as yet (*67*). Castration decreased rat caries in both intact and desalivated rats (*11*). This appeared to eliminate any sex hormone effect on caries mediated *via* the salivary glands. Likewise, Liu (*99*) found a caries increase when mestranol (Enovid), a contraceptive hormone, was injected into female rats, and the caries response was not related to effects on salivary glands. However, in later work, injections of another steroid contraceptive, norethynodrel, also caused caries increases in female rats but these were associated with decreased salivary gland development (*101*). In a further study (*104*), two other contraceptive steroids, ethynlestradiol and medroxyprogesterone acetate, likewise increased caries in female rats, although in this case salivary glands were both inhibited and stimulated by the two agents, respectively. Progesterone, as expected, did not influence caries. Interestingly, Muhler and Shafer (*129*) also noted increased caries in female rats given either estradiol or diethylstilbestrol.

Liu and Lin (*105*) also studied estradiol benzoate and found that caries was increased and salivary glands were underdeveloped in proportion to the dosage levels. In an earlier study, Liu (*100*) described the cariogenic effect of estrogen (estradiol) and noted that while thyroxin given simultaneously did not inhibit caries as it did when given alone, thyroxin apparently permitted normal salivary gland development.

In intact rats fed norethandrolone, an anabolic steroid having only 6% of the androgenic activity of testrosterone, caries was enhanced (*5*); however, in a later study (*6*), rats that were biologically depressed in caries activity by tetracycline administration responded with decreased caries when fed norethandrolone.

It has been reported that adrenalectomy increased dental caries in rats (*144*); however, Sweeney and Shaw (*170*), also studying albino rats, found no significant influence of either adrenalectomy or cortisone injection on caries production.

Recently, Liu and Lin (*102*) observed decreased caries in female rats after adrenalectomy. With increasing hormonal doses, hydrocortisone acetate, caries increased in inverse relation to the degree of salivary enlargement. These workers showed that corticosterone also decreased salivary gland characteristics and increased caries in rats (*103*).

Another pharmacological agent, Diamox (2-acetylamino-1,3,4-thiadiazole-5-sulfonamide), commonly used as a diuretic, caused an increase in caries activity (*80*). No effect was found on salivary pH during the experiment or after 98 days on the treatment. This could have been the indirect result of poor health since the treated animals had severely retarded weight gains.

### *General Discussion*

In any survey of dental caries literature, one is impressed anew with the profound complexity of the caries problem. A major frustration in the search for caries-inhibiting agents has been the lack of correlation between *in vitro* screening and testing procedures and animal caries assays as well as the paucity of satisfactory clinical data with which to compare the *in vitro* and animal studies. Until some basis for establishing such correlations is discovered, it would seem that a multifaceted approach with a variety of *in vitro* and animal studies should and must be continued.

It is unfortunate that enough wide-scale clinical testing of even one organic chemical agent has not been done to establish definitely its anticaries activity, although mild, and the conditions under which it is active. If this were done, the investigator of experimental animal caries would have at least one absolute criterion upon which to design assay procedures consistent with the response in humans. It is reasonable to suppose that a procedure of working backwards from an agent having a known effect on human caries to find a means for demonstrating its activity in animal studies would be successful since the major factors important in human caries, such as microorganisms, fermentable carbohydrate foods, fluoride, salivary flow, and frequency of food intake, have all been demonstrable in animals.

The procedure used to decide which organic chemicals to study in future experiments should be given careful attention. From the findings to date, it appears that biochemicals, whether they be chelators, polyphenols, antioxidants, antibacterial substances, or sources of natural activity such as the seed hull factors, rather than those from the organic chemical shelf, may be the most fruitful source of anticaries factors.

Support for this approach occurs in recent studies by Stralfors (*loc. cit.*), who pursued only meager clues from clinical observations and confirmed the presence of anticaries factors in new plant sources. His work implicates a host of compounds included under the captions of tannins as well as melanoidins and perhaps melanins and caramels found at various steps during the processing of cacao beans, sugar cane, and sugar beets. Finding these new factors in addition to seed hull factors (*loc. cit.*) undoubtedly will stimulate chemists to isolate the responsible compounds.

There is increasing awareness that the agent tested may influence caries indirectly through a physiological or pharmacological effect and in turn, the physiological status of the animal may obscure the influence of the compound tested on caries production (*96, 144*). A change in the frequency of food intake, for example, can influence caries production (*95*) and could, conceivably, be produced by almost any dietary change or supplementation procedure.

The fascinating possibility exists that there is a common denominator for the many and often conflicting data reviewed. The participation in the caries process of organic matrices or macromolecular aggregates on, or attached to, the enamel (within the dental plaque) is generally accepted. Orally occurring minerals or macromolecules either may be components of the matrix or they may catalyze its formation. In a review related to the latter possibility, Siegel (*154*) describes how minerals, in this case the teeth and their accretions, may exhibit pseudo-enzyme activities, especially as oxidases and hydrolases. The oxidation of phenolic compounds is especially noteworthy here since their oxidation is enhanced by polysaccharides, proteins, and other macromolecules easily available in the oral food debris or synthesized by oral microorganisms. Oxidation could proceed with polymerization into lignin-like polymers, or the oxidized compounds could inhibit or modify polymer formation within the organic matrix.

Polyphenols occur widely in plant foods (*13, 166*). The roles of the many naturally occurring sources of anticariogenicity reviewed, especially in seed hulls and chocolate, may be to provide polyphenol precursors, or inhibitors, of polymer formation. The influence on caries has been reviewed for chelators, antioxidants, polyphenols, and various polymers as well as trace metals (reviewed in another chapter). All of these factors could be related to organic polymer formation, or its inhibition, according to the mechanism described by Siegel (*154*). That these factors increase, decrease, or have no effect on caries under different conditions may depend upon their ability to influence polyphenol oxidation or polymer formation. These speculations would explain also the frequent lack of correlation between *in vitro* assays and caries assays since a cariogenic microflora either could be inhibited or favored by the possibilities for polymer formation within the dental plaque.

Peroxidase, discussed as a lactobacillus inhibitor in this review, also plays an especially important role in lignin and, presumably, in "isolignin" formation (*154*). Klinkhamer (*88*) associated dental plaque formation with the stagnated "mobile mucous phase" of saliva. This phase is rich in orogranulocytes containing peroxidase (*89*). The caries-inhibiting and potentiating activities of the peroxidase factors, hydrogen peroxide, and thiocyanate were noted in this review. These observations suggest that a search be made for suitable food additives influencing peroxidase levels or peroxidase-like catalytic activities in the mouth. Sulfites inactivate peroxidases (*13*) and also decrease caries (*73*).

A more general approach would be to search for inhibitors of free radical formation since their formation and utilization in polymer formation from polyphenol oxidation would be likely. Iodine, an obvious free radical inhibitor, was found active in cotton rats fed cariogenic Diet 875, and supplemented with two drops of iodine as Betadine solution two times a day for 4 days. Sixteen days later, caries incidence in water-supplemented controls was 17.5 and in butadiene-supplemented rats was 14.7 ($P < 0.01 > 0.001$) (*114*).

### *Summary*

A host of organic compounds other than those considered elsewhere in this symposium have been assayed for anticaries activity. Many have been studied by microbiological assays or other *in vitro* techniques, fewer by animal studies, and very few by clinical trials.

In most clinical trials, the organic compounds were tested in dentifrices and mouthwashes and appeared to be of no major benefit for caries control. No organic compound among those reviewed has been selected for inclusion in the human diet even though it appears that a number of them, and a number of natural materials as well, have potentials for serving as safe, effective, dietary additives for caries control.

A promising source of anticaries factors is the outer coverings of seeds. These factors have been found in a number of plant species obtained from a wide geographical range. Of these, oat hulls have been studied most; they inhibit both smooth surface and fissure caries produced by a number of different diets in several different assay animals. The crude hulls did not appear toxic or to have any other role when fed than to inhibit caries.

Several seed coats exert a protective effect long after they are removed from the diet. This observation along with microbiological assays indicated that seed coats produce a noncariogenic oral environment. Through chemical separations, phenolic acids and especially polyphenols have been identified in seed coats and possibly may be the active factors. These classes of compounds have been associated with antibacterial, antioxidant, and chelation activities, all of which under particular conditions influence experimental caries.

The hulls also inhibited decalcification of tooth enamel *in vitro*. The identity of the seed hull activity and its mode of action remains to be elucidated, but primarily the activity does not appear inorganic in nature. Recently, brown sugar, molasses, and cacao bean products were found to contain factors that inhibited hamster caries. These findings implicated both inorganic and organic factors. As in seed hulls, polyphenols appeared important. Further testing suggested that tannins and purine derivatives were associated with the anticariogenicity of cocoa and chocolate.

Known compounds tested in both *in vitro* and animal experiments were classified and discussed under the following headings: phenolic acids and polyphenols, antioxidants, antienzymes, carbonyl-binding agents, and complexing agents. Although there were many unexplained and conflicting data, sources of potentially useful activity were found in all categories.

Organic compounds, polymers, and enzymes that may affect the organic film or plaque on tooth surfaces deserve further attention.

Many compounds had physiological and pharmacological activities and affected caries indirectly.

### *Acknowledgment*

The author is grateful to I. J. Wilk for samples of known varieties of rice hulls; to S. Weiss for a purified peanut hull fraction; to B. G. Bibby who provided decalcification values for our hull-containing diets; to Rohm and Haas Co. for enzyme samples; Riviana Foods, Inc., for rice bran samples, and General Mills, Inc., for peroxidase analyses of these samples.

### *Literature Cited*

(1) Albert, A., *Federation Proc.* **1961,** 20 (3), Suppl. 10 Pt. II, 137.
(2) Andlaw, R. J., *J. Dental Res.* **1960**, 39, 1200.
(3) Andlaw, R. J., Bibby, B. G., Buonocore, M. G., *Dental Progr.* **1962,** 3, 36.
(4) Backer-Dirks, O., Kwant, G. W., Starmans, J. L. E. M., *J. Dentistry Belge* **1959,** 50, 163.
(5) Bailey, H. S., Bruno, G. A. *J. Dental Res.* **1965,** 44, 924.
(6) Bailey, H. S., Shaw, S. M., Christian, J. E., *J. Dental Res.* **1964,** 43, 229.
(7) Bartels, H. A., Chiat, L. A., Blechman, H., *J. Dental Res.* **1969,** 48, 1309.
(8) Bate-Smith, E. C., "The Pharmacology of Plant Phenolics," J. W. Fairbairn, Ed., p. 133, Academic, New York, 1959.
(9) Bibby, B. G., "Nutrition and Caries Prevention," Swedish Nutrition Foundation, p. 30, Almquist and Wiksells, Uppsala, 1965.
(10) Bibby, B. G., Weiss, M., *Helv. Odont. Acta* **1967,** 11, 59.
(11) Bixler, D., Muhler, J. C., Shafer, W. G., *J. Dental Res.* **1957**, 36, 709.
(12) Boyers, C. L., Shaw, J. H., Rosenthal, E., Giordano, R., *J. Dental Res.* **1963,** 42, 1517.
(13) Braverman, J. B. S., "Introduction to the Biochemistry of Foods," p. 294, Elsevier, New York, 1963.
(14) Brunel, A. L., Causeret, J., Houssiaux, C., Hugot, D., *Bull. Groupe Intern. Rech. Sci. Stomatol.* **1966,** 2, 157.
(15) *Ibid.,* **1966,** 3, 267.
(16) Busta, F. F., Speck, M. L., *Appl. Microbiol.* **1968,** 18, 424.
(17) Buttner, W., Muhler, J. C., *J. Dental Res.* **1959,** 38, 823.
(18) Cathcart, W. H., Merz, A., *Food Res.* **1942,** 7, 96.
(19) Cerul, D. M., Manley, R. S., Frager, M., Manly, P. C., *J. Oral Therap. Pharmacol.* **1965**, 1, 501.
(20) Chatt, E. M., "Cocoa," p. 149, Interscience, New York, 1953.
(21) Chenoweth, M. B., *Pharmacol. Rev.* **1956,** 8, 57.
(22) Cherhausek, D. S., Mitchell, D. F., *J. Dental Res.* **1951,** 30, 393.
(23) Cherhausek, D. S., Mitchell, D. F., *Science* **1950,** 112, 273.
(24) Clarkson, B. H., Bibby, B. G., *J. Dental Res.* **1969,** 48, 916.
(25) Constant, M. A., Phillips, P. H., Elvehjem, C. A., *J. Nutr.* **1952,** 46, 271.

(26) Constant, M. A., Sievert, H. W., Phillips, P. H., Elvehjem, C. A., *J. Nutr.* **1954,** 53, 17.
(27) Dogon, I. L., Amdur, B. H., "Program and Abstracts of Papers," p. 54, International Association for Dental Research, Chicago, 1966.
(28) Dogon, I. L., Kerr, A. C., Amdur, B. H., *Arch. Oral Biol.* **1962**, 7, 81.
(29) Dreizen, S., Mann, A. W., Spies, T. D., Carson, B. C., Cline, J. K., *J. Dental Res.* **1947,** 26, 93.
(30) Dubois-Prevost, R., *Hygie* **1961,** 17, 8.
(31) Dunning, J. M., Hodge, A. T., "Program and Abstracts of Papers," p. 166, International Association for Dental Research, New York, 1970.
(32) Eigen, E., Donohue, J. J., King, W. J., Weiss, S., "Program and Abstracts of Papers," p. 108, International Association for Dental Research, Chicago, 1963.
(33) *Federation Proc.* **1961,** 20 (3), Suppl. 10, Pt. II.
(34) Finn, S. B., Jamison, H. C., *J. Dentistry Children* **1963,** 30, 17.
(35) Foreman, H., Vier, M., Magee, M., *J. Biol. Chem.* **1953,** 203, 1045.
(36) Forscher, B. K., Hess, W. C., *J. Am. Dental Assoc.* **1954,** 48, 134.
(37) Fosdick, L. S., *Science* **1956,** 123, 988.
(38) Fosdick, L. S., Calandra, J. C., *J. Dental Res.* **1947,** 26, 309.
(39) Fosdick, L. S., Calandra, J. C., Blackwell, R. Q., Burrill, J. H., *J. Dental Res.* **1953,** 32, 486.
(40) Francis, M. D., Meckel, A. H., *J. Dental Res.* **1960,** 39, 697.
(41) Frasher, L. A., Hein, J. W., *J. Dental Res.* **1958,** 37, 75.
(42) Fuller, J. E., Mueller, W. S., Swanson, *J. Dairy Sci.* **1942,** 25, 883.
(43) Geczik, R., King, W. J., "Abstracts of the Fortieth General Meeting," p. 62, International Association for Dental Research, Chicago, 1961.
(44) Geller, J. H., Rovelstad, G. H., *J. Dental Res.* **1959,** 38, 1060.
(45) Gibbons, R. J., *J. Dental Res.* **1968,** 47, 926.
(46) Gillings, B., *J. Dental Res.* **1963,** 42, 8.
(47) Giordano, R. A., Shaw, J. H., *J. Dental Res.* **1962,** 41, 96.
(48) Goose, D. H., Hartles, R. L., "Principles of Preventive Dentistry," p. 25, Macmillan, New York, 1964.
(49) Gray, J. A., Francis, M. D., Griebstein, W. J., *In* "Chemistry and Prevention of Dental Caries," p. 164, Thomas, Springfield, Ill., 1962.
(50) Green, G. H., *J. Dental Res.* **1960,** 39, 699.
(51) Grenby, T. H., *Arch. Oral Biol.* **1967,** 12, 513.
(52) *Ibid.,* **1967,** 12, 523.
(53) *Ibid.,* **1967,** 12, 531.
(54) Grippaudo, G., Valfre, F., Santa Catterina, G., Cecchetti, G., *Ann. Stomatol. (Roma)* **1966,** 15, 867.
(55) Gustafsson, B. E., Krasse, B., *Acta Odontol. Scand.* **1958,** 16, 355.
(56) Gustafsson, B. E., Quensel, C. E., Swenander-Lanke, L., Lundquist, C., Grahnen, H., Bonow, B. E., Krasse, B., *Acta Odontol. Scand.* **1954,** 11, 232.
(57) Haldi, J., Wynn, W., Law, M. L., *J. Dental Res.* **1962,** 41, 398.
(58) Haldi, J., Wynn, W., Law, M. L., Tyler, T., *J. Dental Res.* **1960,** 39, 530.
(59) Hawes, R. R., Bibby, B. G., *J. Am. Dental Assoc.* **1953,** 46, 280.
(60) Hayden, J., Glass, R. L., *J. Dental Res.* **1959,** 38, 671.
(61) Hein, J. W., "Advances in Experimental Caries Research," R. F. Sognnaes, Ed., p. 197, Waverly, Baltimore, 1955.
(62) Hendershot, L. C., Mansell, R. E., Forsaith, J., "Metal-Binding in Medicine," M. J. Seven and L. A. Johnson, Eds., p. 306, Lippincott, Philadelphia, 1960.
(63) Irwin, M., Leaver, A. G., Walsh, J. P., *J. Dental Res.* **1951,** 36, 166.
(64) Ishi, T., Konig, K. G., Muhlemann, H. R., *Helv. Odontol. Acta* **1968,** 12, 41.

(65) Ishikawa, T., *Shikwa Gakuho* **1968,** 68, 56.
(66) Iwamoto, Y., Nakamura, R., Tsunemitsu, A., Matsumura, T., *Arch. Oral Biol.* **1968,** 13, 1015.
(67) Jenkins, G. N., "Chemistry and Prevention of Dental Caries," R. F. Sognnaes, Ed., p. 126, Thomas, Springfield, Ill., 1962.
(68) Jenkins, G. N., "Nutrition and Caries Prevention," Swedish Nutrition Foundation, p. 67, Almqvist and Wiksells, Uppsala, 1965.
(69) Jenkins, G. N., Smales, F. C., *Arch. Oral Biol.* **1966,** 11, 599.
(70) Jenkins, G. N., Forster, M. G., Speirs, R. L., Kleinberg, I., *Brit. Dental J.* **1959,** 106, 195.
(71) Jordan, H. V., Bowler, A. E., Berger, N. D., *J. Dental Res.* **1961,** 40, 199.
(72) Jordan, H. V., Fitzgerald, R. J., Berger, N. D., *J. Dental Res.* **1961**, 40, 878.
(73) *Ibid.*, **1962,** 41, 61.
(74) Jordan, H. V., Fitzgerald, R. J., Bowler, A. E., *J. Dental Res.* **1960,** 39, 116.
(75) Jordan, H. V., Zipkin, I., Fitzgerald, R. J., Berger, N. D., *J. Dental Res.* **1964,** 43, 3.
(76) Kamo, T., *Japan. J. Dental Health* **1967,** 17, 139.
(77) Kardachi, B. J. R., *J. Dental Res.* **1967,** 46, 1308.
(78) Kempf, N. W., "The Technology of Chocolate," p. 31–32, 46, 54, Manufacturing Confectioner Publ. Co., Oak Park, Ill., 1964.
(79) Kesel, R. G., O'Donnell, J. F., Wallace, D. A., *J. Am. Dental Assoc.* **1954,** 48, 8.
(80) Keyes, P. H., *Arch. Oral Biol.* **1960**, 1, 304.
(81) Keyes, P. H., *J. Dental Res.* **1946**, 25, 469.
(82) *Ibid.*, **1958,** 37, 1077.
(83) Keyes, P. H., White, C. L., *J. Am. Dental Assoc.* **1959,** 58, 43.
(84) Keyes, P. H., Fitzgerald, R. J., Jordan, H. V., "Abstracts of the Fortieth General Meeting," p. 62, International Association for Dental Research, Chicago, 1962.
(85) Kinkel, H. J., Cremer, H. D., *J. Dental Res.* **1960,** 39, 640.
(86) Kinkel, H. J., Newiger, J., *Deut. Zahnnaerztl. Z.* **1960,** 15, 1083.
(87) Klebanoff, S. J., Luebke, R. G., *Proc. Soc. Exptl. Biol. Med.* **1965,** 118, 483.
(88) Klinkhamer, J. M., "Dental Biochemistry," E. P. Lazzari, Ed., p. 137, Lea and Febiger, Philadelphia, 1968.
(89) Klinkhamer, J. M., "Program and Abstract of Papers," p. 168, International Association for Dental Research, New York, 1970.
(90) Konig, K. G., Grenby, T. H., *Arch. Oral Biol.* **1965**, 10, 143.
(91) Konig, K. G., Muhlemann, H. R., *Helv. Odontol. Acta* **1964,** 8, 22.
(92) Konig, K. G., Muhlemann, H. R., *Arch. Oral Biol.* **1967,** 12, 1297.
(93) Konig, K. G., Marthaler, T. M., Muhlemann, H. R., *Arch. Oral Biol.* **1961**, 3, 258.
(94) Kyes, F. M., Overton, N. J., McKean, T. W., *J. Am. Dental Assoc.* **1961,** 63, 189.
(95) Larson, R. H., Rubin, M., Zipkin, I., *Arch. Oral Biol.* **1962**, 7, 463.
(96) Larson, R. H., Zipkin, I., Rubin, M., *Arch. Oral Biol.* **1961,** 5, 49.
(97) Limbasuta, S., Singh, B., Johansen, E., *J. Dental Res.* **1961**, 40, 658.
(98) Lisanti, V. F., Eichel, H., *J. Dental Res.* **1963,** 42, 1030.
(99) Liu, F. T. Y., Lofgren, R., Hoots, I., *J. Dental Res.* **1966,** 45, 1236.
(100) Liu, F. T. Y., *J. Dental Res.* **1967,** 46, 471.
(101) *Ibid.*, **1968,** 48, 1047.
(102) Liu, F. T. Y., Lin, H. S., *J. Dental Res.* **1968,** 47, 158.
(103) *Ibid.*, **1969,** 48, 467.
(104) *Ibid.*, **1969**, 48, 477.
(105) Liu, F. T. Y., Lin, H. S., Zullo, T. G., *J. Dental Res.* **1969,** 48, 485.

(106) Ludwig, T. G., Taylor, W. G., *N. Z. Dental J.* **1957,** 53, 63.
(107) Lundquist, C., *J. Dental Res.* **1951,** 30, 203.
(108) Madsen, K. O., Thesis, University of Wisconsin, Madison, 1958.
(109) Madsen, K. O., Edmonds, E. J., *Arch. Oral Biol.* **1964,** 9, 209.
(110) Madsen, K. O., Edmonds, E. J., *J. Dental Res.* **1962,** 41, 405.
(111) *Ibid.,* **1963,** 42, 137.
(112) *Ibid.,* **1963,** 42, 867.
(113) *Ibid.,* **1964,** 43, 860.
(114) Madsen, K. O., Edmonds, E. J., unpublished data.
(115) Mahler, I. R., Manly, R. S., *J. Am. Dental Assoc.* **1958,** 56, 854.
(116) Martell, A. E., "Metal-Binding in Medicine," M. J. Seven and L. A. Johnson, Eds., p. 257, Lippincott, Philadelphia, 1960.
(117) Masuda, Y., Sasaki, H., Yoshioka, Y., Hara, K., Goto, K., *J. Osaka Dental Univ.* **1968,** 21, 116.
(118) McClure, F. J., *Arch. Oral Biol.* **1964,** 9, 219.
(119) McClure, F. J., *J. Dental Res.* **1948,** 27, 34.
(120) *Ibid.,* **1963,** 42, 693.
(121) McClure, F. J., *Public Health Rept.* **1949,** 64, 1061.
(122) McClure, F. J., *Science* **1964,** 144, 1337.
(123) Morioka, T., Saj, S., Inoue, M., Matsumura, T., *Arch. Oral Biol.* **1969,** 14, 549.
(124) Morrison, M., Steele, W. F., "Biology of the Mouth," P. Person, Ed., p. 89, King, Baltimore, 1968.
(125) Mosimann, G., *Intern. Chocolate Rev.* **1947,** 2, 186.
(126) Muhlemann, H. R., Konig, K. G., *Helv. Odontol. Acta* **1962,** 6, 33.
(127) *Ibid.,* **1967,** 11, 152.
(128) Muhlemann, H. R., Meyer, R. W., Konig, K. G., Marthaler, T. M., *Helv. Odontol. Acta* **1961,** 5, 18.
(129) Muhler, J. C., Shafer, W. G., *J. Dental Res.* **1955,** 34, 661.
(130) *Ibid.,* **1959,** 38, 795.
(131) Muhler, J. C., Bixler, D., Shafer, W. G., *J. Dental Res.* **1957,** 36, 883.
(132) Muhler, J. C., Shafer, W. G., Clark, P., *J. Dental Res.* **1963,** 42, 768.
(133) Neuberg, C., Reinfurth, E., *Biochem. Z.* **1918,** 98, 365.
(134) Nizel, A. E., Harris, R. S., *J. Dental Res.* **1964,** 43, 1123.
(135) *Nutr. Rev.* **1962,** 20, 272.
(136) *Ibid.,* **1965,** 23, 168.
(137) Osborn, T. W. B., Noriskin, J. N., Staz, J., *J. Dental Res.* **1937,** 16, 545.
(138) Poe, C. F., Johnson, C. C., *Acta Pharm. Tox. Kbh.* **1953,** 9, 267.
(139) Regolati, B., Konig, K. G., Muhlemann, H. R., *Helv. Odontol. Acta* **1969,** 13, 28.
(140) Rozeik, F., Cremer, H. D., Hannover, R., *Deut. Zahnnaerztl. Z.* **1956,** 11, 1104.
(141) Salazar, V., Harris, R. S., Nizel, A. E., *in* "Program and Abstracts of Papers," p. 88, International Association for Dental Research, Chicago, 1965.
(142) Schrauffstater, E., *Experientia* **1948,** 4, 484.
(143) Seven, M. J., Johnson, L. A., "Metal-Binding in Medicine," Lippincott, Philadelphia, 1960.
(144) Shafer, W. G., Muhler, J. C., "Advances in Experimental Caries Research," R. F. Sognnaes, Ed., p. 137, Waverly, Baltimore, 1955.
(145) Shapiro, M., Brat, V., Ershoff, B. H., *J. Dental Res.* **1960,** 39, 332.
(146) Shaw, J. H., "Chemistry and Prevention of Dental Caries," R. S. Sognnaes, Ed., p. 180, Thomas, Springfield, Ill., 1962.
(147) Shaw, J. H., *J. Dental Res.* **1950,** 29, 23.
(148) Shaw, J. H., *J. Nutr.* **1954,** 54, 177.
(149) Shaw, J. H., *Pharmacol. Rev.* **1959,** 11, 705.
(150) Shaw, J. H., Griffiths, D., *J. Dental Res.* **1960,** 39, 377.

(151) *Ibid.*, **1963**, 42, 1004.
(152) Shaw, J. H., Ensfield, B. J., Wollman, D. H., *J. Nutr.* **1959**, 67, 253.
(153) Shaw, J. H., Schweigert, B. S., McIntire, J. M., Elvehjem, C. A., Phillips, P. H., *J. Nutr.* **1944**, 28, 333.
(154) Siegel, S. M., "Biology of the Mouth," P. Person, Ed., p. 111, King, Baltimore, 1968.
(155) Smales, F. C., *J. Dental Res.* **1963**, 42, 1103.
(156) Soni, N. N., Bibby, B. G., *J. Dental Res.* **1961**, 40, 185.
(157) Stephan, R. M., *Science* **1940**, 92, 578.
(158) Stephan, R. M., Harris, M. R., "Advances in Experimental Caries Research," R. F. Sognnaes, Ed., p. 47, Waverly, Baltimore, 1955.
(159) Stephan, R. M., Miller, B. F., *Proc. Soc. Exptl. Biol. Med.* **1944**, 55, 101.
(160) Stralfors, A., *Arch. Oral Biol.* **1966**, 11, 149.
(161) *Ibid.*, **1966**, 11, 323.
(162) *Ibid.*, **1966**, 11, 609.
(163) *Ibid.*, **1966**, 11, 617.
(164) *Ibid.*, **1967**, 12, 321.
(165) *Ibid.*, **1967**, 12, 959.
(166) *Ibid.*, **1967**, 12, 1375.
(167) Stralfors, A., Thilander, H., Bergenholtz, A., *Arch. Oral Biol.* **1967**, 12, 1367.
(168) Sulser, G. F., Fosket, R. R., Foskick, L. S., *J. Am. Dental Assoc.* **1958**, 56, 368.
(169) Sweeney, E. A., Shaw, J. H., *Arch. Oral Biol.* **1963**, 8, 775.
(170) Sweeney, E. A., Shaw, J. H., *J. Dental Res.* **1965**, 44, 96.
(171) *Ibid.*, **1965**, 44, 973.
(172) Taketa, F., Phillips, P. H., *J. Am. Dietet. Assoc.* **1957**, 33, 575.
(173) Thompson, D. T., Vogel, J. J., Phillips, P. H., *J. Dental Res.* **1965**, 44, 596.
(174) Vogel, J. J., Thompson, D. J., Phillips, P. H., *J. Dental Res.* **1962**, 41, 707.
(175) Wallace, D. A., *Dental Progr.* **1962**, 2, 242.
(176) Walsh, J. P., Green, R. W., *J. Dental Res.* **1950**, 29, 270.
(177) Zachterl, W. A., "Program and Abstracts of Papers," p. 133, International Association for Dental Research, New York, 1970.
(178) Zipkin, I., *Proc. Soc. Exptl. Biol. Med.* **1953**, 82, 80.
(179) Zipkin, I., McClure, F. J., *J. Am. Dental Assoc.* **1957**, 55, 15.
(180) Zipkin, I., McClure, F. J., *Proc. Soc. Exptl. Biol. Med.* **1958**, 97, 318.

RECEIVED August 14, 1968. This research was supported in part by a USPHS research grant DE-01555 from the National Institute of Dental Research, National Institutes of Health, Bethesda, Md., and in part by Medical Research Foundation of Texas, Houston.

# 7

# Minerals: Fluorine and Dental Caries

HAROLD C. HODGE and FRANK A. SMITH

University of Rochester School of Medicine and Dentistry,
Rochester, N.Y. 14620

*Sources of fluoride entering the body by food and beverages are described. Total daily dietary fluoride in various countries ranges between 0.2 and 2.7 mg. In the U.S., the range appears to be 0.3–0.8 mg per day. Absorbed fluoride ion is transported in the blood in both exchangeable and bound forms. No soft tissues store fluoride other than in sites of ectopic calcification. Excretion of absorbed fluoride is chiefly by way of the urine, 90–95% of the total excreted fluoride. That fluoride retained in the body is found almost entirely in the bone. Levels of skeletal fluoride are related to the levels of fluoride found in drinking water and to age. Reduction in caries incidence by fluoride in various vehicles is reviewed.*

The ubiquitous nature of fluorine is nowhere better illustrated than by its existence in detectable traces in virtually every item of the normal diet of man all over the world. Fluoride, thirteenth in abundance among the elements, constitutes about 0.078% of the earth's crust—slightly greater than the chloride content, 0.055%. The principal fluoride minerals are fluorspar (calcium fluoride), cryolite (sodium aluminum fluoride), and a large number of fluoride-substituted minerals—*e.g.*, fluorapatite, fluorocarbonates, fluorophosphates, and the fluorosilicates. One means of disseminating fluorides throughout the world has been volcanic action, in which huge amounts of HF may be emitted. Nommik (78) cites the estimate that 135,000 tons of HF are discharged annually from the volcanoes in the Katmai area of Alaska alone. Modern processing of rock phosphate, a multimillion ton industry and an important source of fluoride dispersion, has helped to control fluoride emission in certain areas. The superphosphate industry in Florida, for example, by scrubbing fluorides from the effluents, recovers most of that released in the acid process. Bredeman (*8*) reviewed the geochemistry of fluorine. Fluoride rocks in general are highly variable in their fluoride contents and, as would be expected, the fluoride content of soils reflects the nature of the mineral components. Nommik (*78*) found that sandy soils in Sweden usually contained lower concentrations of fluoride than clay soils. The well waters in these areas reflected the soil fluoride concentrations and, to a lesser degree, so did the vegetation. Several-fold variations were found in the fluoride concentrations of different cereals raised on the same farm (*78*).

Some plants are characteristically rich in fluoride; most contain only trace amounts. It seems reasonable to assume that the inorganic fluoride in plants has been picked up by the roots from fluoride ion in soil waters. The camellia family is famous for its ability to concentrate fluoride; dried tea leaves frequently contain several hundred parts per million F. Plant materials have not been as intensively nor as widely studied as have animal tissues, perhaps (as Nommik points out) because there is no known function for fluoride in plants, and with a few notable exceptions only trace amounts occur. Roots appear to contain more than stalks, which in turn contain more than seeds. Husks have larger concentrations than do the inner parts of seeds or tubers; *e.g.*, in flour milling, fluoride is most abundant in the seed husks (*78*) and least in the inner parts of the grain. Peeled potatoes contain only 0.07 to 0.25 ppm F, whereas the peelings range from 0.5 to 0.8 ppm (*85*). Although the nature of the fluoride in plant material has not been elucidated completely, most (about 80% or sometimes more) of the fluoride is leached easily into aqueous extracts and therefore presumably occurs as a simple inorganic fluoride. All plant fluoride is considered inorganic, with the exception of that in a few species of plants of the *Dichapetalum* genus native to the Transvaal or to West Africa, of the *Acacia* from Australia, and of the *Palicourea* from Brazil, which contain an organic fluoride, either fluoroacetate or a longer chain fluoro fatty acid (*47, 79, 80*). Certain bacteria can cleave the fluorocarbon bond (*34*).

The process of leaching into soil water ultimately makes fluoride available in well waters for human consumption; a major source in parts of the United States is fluoride carried long distances in deep subterranean streams (*75*). The disfiguring effects of excess fluorides on the teeth and the instances of skeletal fluorosis have prompted many surveys of water fluoride concentrations. The beneficial effect on tooth health of small concentrations of fluoride in community water supplies has recently been another reason for natural water fluoride surveys. Most water supplies have only trace amounts of fluoride (less than 0.1 ppm); in widely distributed areas around the surface of the earth, however, some well waters contain from 0.5 ppm to 10 or rarely 20 or more ppm F. Deeper wells often have higher fluoride concentrations than shallow wells.

In the United States today about 10,000,000 persons drink waters naturally fluoridated at concentrations of 0.7 ppm or more. It is estimated that the water supplies of approximately 4,000,000 persons contain "excessive" levels—*i.e.*, above the optimal range of 0.7–1.2 ppm (*45, 82*). In addition, nearly 62,000,000 residents drink fluoridated community water supplies (*45, 82*).

### *Human Diet*

The fluoride consumed in the diet is small and relatively constant in amount. In eight countries in Asia, Europe, and North America where daily dietary fluoride consumption has been estimated, at least 0.2 mg F is consumed in each country, and in only three is the consumption from food greater than 1 mg daily (Table I). In the areas where the diet analyses were made, water fluoride concentrations have been low without exception. Certain foods cooked in fluoridated water tend to increase in fluoride content (*68*).

**Table I. Daily Dietary Fluoride**[a]

| *Country* | *Mg F Ingested in Food and Water* | *Ppm F in Drinking Water* | *Reference* |
|---|---|---|---|
| Canada | 0.18–0.3 | 0.1 | *36* |
| England | 0.3–0.5 | trace | *65* |
| Japan | 0.47–2.66[b] | 0.01–0.08[c] | *50* |
| Newfoundland | 2.74[d] | trace | *22* |
| Norway | 0.22–0.31 | 0.01–0.07 | *15* |
| Russia | 0.6–1.2 | 0.2–0.3 | *30* |
| Sweden | 0.9 | | *1* |
| Switzerland | 0.5[e] | | *26* |
| U.S.A. | 0.2–0.3[e] | | *4, 70* |
| | 0.34–0.80 | 0.1 | *42* |

[a] After Cholak (*13*); cf Osis *et al.* (*81*).
[b] Including 0.07–0.86 mg from green tea.
[c] Mg F ingested.
[d] Including 1 mg from tea.
[e] Exclusive of that in drinking water.

The major categories of foods (Table II) contain traces or more of F (*13, 26, 70*). Thus, recent analyses of meats show only a few ppm F at most. Sea foods have special interest because sea water contains 1–1.4 ppm F. Fish meat without bone or skin has been reported several times to contain about 1 ppm F. Sardines as consumed, however, may contain

**Table II. Fluoride Concentration (PPM) in Fresh Foods**

| *Food* | *Data to 1959 From Cholak* (13) | *Recent Data* | *Reference* |
|---|---|---|---|
| Meats | 0.01–7.7 | 0.14–2 | *15, 50, 60, 88* |
| Fish | <0.10–24 | 1.0– | *15, 50, 58, 60, 88* |
| Sardines | | 8–40 | *15* |
| Shrimp | | 50[a] | *15* |
| Fish meal | | 186 | |
| Citrus fruits | 0.04–0.36 | 0.07–0.17 | *2, 35* |
| Noncitrus fruits | 0.02–1.32 | 0.03–0.84 | *2, 15, 35, 50* |
| Cereals and cereal products | <0.10–20 | 0.18–2.8 | *15, 35, 50, 58, 60, 83, 88, 91* |
| Vegetables and tubers | 0.10–3.0 | 0.02–0.9 | *2, 15, 35, 50, 60, 83, 88, 91* |

[a] Shrimp meat, 0.4 ppm; shrimp shell, 18–48 ppm (*72, 93*).

as much as 40 ppm. The newly developed protein source, fish meal, may contain 186 ppm (one analysis); 100 grams of this fish meal would contribute nearly 20 mg of F to the diet. Japanese shrimp was reported to contain as much as 50 ppm; however, Smith and Gardner (*93*) found 0.2–0.4 ppm in United States shrimp flesh and 18–48 ppm in the shell. Bone contains much more fluoride (values of 200–1000 ppm are not unusual) than meat, so that fish eaten bones and all—sardines, for example —contain relatively high concentrations.

Citrus and noncitrus fruits are low in fluorides—less than 1 ppm. In older analyses, an occasional reported high value may show only a failure to take precautions against contamination by fluoride insecticides. Cereals and cereal products usually contain only a few ppm at most, and vegetables and tubers probably about 1 ppm, although up to 3 ppm has been reported. Unless a diet contains substantial amounts of some of the sea foods or tea, dietary fluorides always will be low.

Fluoride ingested in fluids in many parts of the world can be traced to the fluoride naturally present in the drinking water, or, particularly in the United States, to fluoride added in community fluoridation projects. Beverages, with the exception of tea, are not important contributors of fluoride (Table III). A few wines contain up to 6 ppm, but most less than 1 ppm.

One of the best-studied sources of fluoride in the human diet is tea. Tea infusions on the average contain about 1 ppm (*65*); instant tea, somewhat less. Most of the fluoride in bulk tea is extractable. The early work of Reid (*86*), and of Lawrenz and Mitchell (*62*), who calculated that green tea fluoride was only about 5% less well assimilated than was sodium fluoride in the diet of rats, has been borne out by more recent studies. Zimmerman (*106*) showed that 60–70% of the fluoride in tea leaves could be removed by steeping or boiling for a few minutes, and Quenton (*85*) found that 86–92% of the tea fluoride was extractable. Fresh coffee bean contains up to 1.6 ppm; the decoction must be dilute indeed. If 2 grams of instant coffee (1.7 ppm) are used per cup, the F concentration will be only 0.02 ppm in this beverage. Milk usually has about 0.1 ppm, although a few higher values have been recorded. The available analyses for Coca Cola and for orange juice are quite low; if a fluoridated water supply is used to prepare these drinks, the resulting F concentrations, of course, would reflect that of the water supply.

Since water-borne fluorides exceed 1 ppm in certain localities, in these neighborhoods water fluoride would be the principal source of F ingestion.

How important water can be as a source is shown from Largent's (*61*) careful balance studies of adults, aged 30 to 57 years, who had long resided in their communities, and whose fluoride intake and output were

**Table III. Fluoride in Beverages**

| *Beverage* | *Ppm F* | *Reference* |
|---|---|---|
| Wine | 0.0–6.3 | *13* |
| Beer | 0.15–0.86 | *13* |
| Tea infusion | 0.1–2.0 | *50, 106* |
| Instant (soln.) | 0.2 | *106* |
| Coffee bean | 0.2–1.6 | *13* |
| Instant (powder) | 1.7 | *100* |
| Milk | 0.04–0.55 | *13* |
| Coca Cola | 0.07 | *13* |
| Orange juice | 0.0–0.05 | *39* |

**Table IV. Relation of Fluoride Ingested to that in Water and Food Consumed**[a]

| *Ppm F in Water* | *Age* | *Res., Yrs.* | *Days Obsd.* | *Daily Intake, Mg F* | | |
|---|---|---|---|---|---|---|
| | | | | *Fluid* | *Food* | *Sum* |
| <0.1 | 33 | 8 | 140 | 0.3 | 0.2 | 0.5 |
| 1[b] | | | | | | |
| 2 | 35 | 10 | 96 | 2.4 | 1.2 | 3.6 |
| 5.5 | 55 | 29 | 60 | 3.8 | 1.3 | 5.1 |
| 6.1 | 57 | 34 | 133 | 6.7 | 1.0 | 7.7 |
| 8 | 57 | 19 | 140 | 11.3 | 2.5 | 13.8 |
| 20 | 30 | 8 | 45 | 20.8 | 1.5 | 22.3 |

[a] Adapted from Largent (*61*).
[b] Comparable data could not be found for individuals consuming water containing 1 ppm F.

estimated daily for periods of 45 to 140 days. The food fluoride usually totaled about 1.5 mg F or less, regardless of the fluoride concentration in the drinking water (Table IV). In contrast, the fluoride consumed in fluids depends notably on the water concentration and reflects the fact that the average individual drinks about a liter of water per day. Thus, the total fluoride intake (in mg F) reflects almost numerically the water fluoride concentration (in ppm) in any community.

Although the benefits of fluoride in dental health are unquestioned and the possible usefulness in certain metabolic bone disorders is under study, no convincing demonstration has been made of the essentiality of fluoride in growth and reproduction.

A summary of the interrelations of certain vitamins, especially vitamin C and vitamin D, and fluoride has been prepared by Suttie and Phillips (*96*).

In summary, diets are usually low in F and remarkably uniform world-round (0.5–1.5 mg/day). Most items of food except bone and most beverages except tea contain small concentrations of F. Water-borne fluorides are variable in concentration and, if elevated, constitute the principal source of F intake.

### *Fluoride Metabolism*

The metabolism of inorganic fluoride is reviewed under four headings: considerations of the absorption of fluoride in the gastrointestinal tract, its patterns and rates of distribution through the body following absorption, the modes, quantities, and rates of excretion, and the importance of the skeleton and other calcified tissues as deposition sites (*43*; *46*, p. 517).

**Absorption.** Only fluoride ion (from practically all inorganic sources; organic fluorides are not considered here) reaches the blood stream, regardless of the form in which fluoride is taken into the body. The percentage of fluoride absorbed depends principally on the solubility of the compound. Ingested soluble fluorides—*e.g.*, a dilute solution of sodium fluoride, sodium fluorosilicate, or HF—probably yield nearly 100% of the fluoride to the circulation. With less soluble materials, such as calcium fluoride, sodium aluminum fluoride, or bone, the absorption is less. Thus, one-third to two-thirds of the fluoride in bone meal can be accounted for in the urine. Fluoride in milk is absorbed more slowly but with about the same efficiency as the same amount in water (*23*).

Some fluoride is absorbed from the stomach, perhaps because the relatively undissociated HF molecule can penetrate the mucosal membrane. Extremely rapid absorption occurs in the gut; analyses of the contents of the GI tract (rat) show that approximately half of a small dose of sodium fluoride is absorbed in 30 minutes and 90% in an hour and a half.

**Distribution.** The total normal blood fluoride concentration usually lies in the range from 0.10 to 0.15 ppm. About 75% of this fluoride is carried in the plasma, the balance in or on the red blood cells. Most of the human serum fluoride (about 90%) can be called "nonexchangeable" or "bound" fluoride, because it accompanies albumin when the serum components are separated electrophoretically (*98*). The concentration of exchangeable fluoride—*i.e.*, fluoride ion—in the serum of individuals drinking nonfluoridated water lies in the range 0.004–0.008 ppm; of individuals drinking fluoridated water (1 ppm) the range is 0.01–0.02 ppm (*92, 99*). Less than 5% of radiofluoride added to dog plasma was bound and not ultrafilterable under physiologic conditions (*12;* compare *89*). Distribution is rapid following an oral dose of fluoride; blood concentrations peak in an hour or less and thereafter rapidly decline, so that in 4 hours serum concentrations are again near normal. Given intravenously, fluoride concentrations fall very rapidly for 2 or 3 minutes (probably the mixing time for fluoride throughout the circulating blood); thereafter, evidence of a slower process appears with a half-time of 30 minutes (probably skeletal deposition); a much slower process then ensues, with a half-time of 2 or 3 hours (probably kidney excretion). The organs and soft tissues in general exhibit fluoride concentrations (as shown by radiofluoride studies) paralleling but slightly less than blood concentrations at the same time. Fluoride distribution is much like that of chloride, except somewhat slower. Tosteson (*102*), using red blood cells marked with $^{18}F$, measured the rapid movement of $^{18}F$ from the cells into nonlabelled medium; the transfer was a first-order reaction. The $^{18}F$ cell-to-medium ratio was 0.50; a small and variable fraction of the cell fluoride was rapidly exchangeable, perhaps indicating some membrane binding of fluoride. Comparative studies with $^{38}Cl$ showed almost exactly the same cell-to-medium ratio (0.54) with no evidence of a rapidly exchangeable cell fraction. The rate of removal of chloride from the cell was also exponential. The outflow rate constants were 0.3 per second for $^{18}F$ and 3.1 per second for $^{38}Cl$. The flux as measured in micro-micromoles per square centimeter per second was 2300 for $^{18}F$ and 13,100 for $^{38}Cl$. The membrane transport of fluoride may thus be described as a passive process analogous to but quantitatively slower than the transport of chloride.

No soft tissue stores fluoride. Any ectopic calcification, however, fixes fluoride; thus, certain tissues that often contain calcified loci, such as the aorta and the placenta, may show elevated F contents. For example, with age, both calcium and fluoride contents increase in the aorta. The fluoride concentrations in many tissues (muscle, liver, heart, etc.) lie in the range of 0.1 to perhaps 2 or 3 ppm. The normal concentrations in milk are almost equivalent to those in blood, about 0.1 ppm; saliva also contains about 0.1 ppm. Questions often arise about the thyroid, perhaps because fluoride is a halogen and the thyroid has such extraordinary ability to fix and hold another halogen, iodine. Fluoride is not stored in the thyroid, and injected $^{18}F$ rises in the thyroid only to a concentration near that in blood. When radiofluoride is given to a pregnant animal or woman, the placenta also seems to act as somewhat of a barrier, in that $^{18}F$ in the fetal blood stream does not reach the same concentration as in the maternal blood stream; the placenta concentration is intermediate (Figure 1). Fetal blood F concentrations (measured chemically) are usually about 0.1 ppm, or approximately the same as those in the maternal circulation. A few high values for placental fluoride can be attributed to ectopic calcifications. Any deposit of calcium phosphate has strong powers for fixing fluoride. The human aorta also sometimes contains elevated amounts of fluoride. Samples taken from individuals whose drinking water supplies had contained up to 4 ppm showed no relation between aorta F and drinking water F. With increasing age, however, the fluoride concentration of the aortas tended to increase. Aorta calcium also tends to increase with age; Call *et al.* (*11*) showed a linear relation between fluoride concentrations and calcium concentrations in

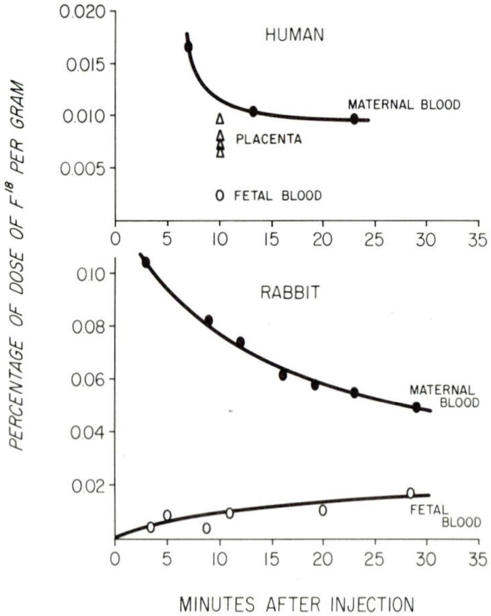


*Figure 1. Maternal-fetal transfer of* $^{18}F$ *in the human and in the rabbit* (25)

samples of aorta. Urinary calculi also fixed fluoride if they contained calcium phosphate.

**Excretion.** Ordinarily, the urine is the principal route of excretion of fluoride (*48*). Table V shows that urinary fluorides ordinarily constitute 90–95% of the total excreted in the feces and in the urine. Fecal excretion frequently is 5–10% of the total; some of this may be unabsorbed fluoride; some of it almost certainly is fluoride that has been absorbed and then re-excreted into the gut by the various digestive juices. The sweat may constitute a significant route of excretion. There are few data which indicate how much fluoride is lost through the sweat under what might be considered comfortable conditions of temperature and humidity. Under conditions of extreme sweating, as much as a third of a small dose of fluoride has been recovered in the sweat. This route may be highly important for persons in hot climates who consume large quantities of fluoridated water. Small amounts of fluoride are laid down in the skin, deposited in hair, and removed in this way from the body; these routes are almost certainly unimportant.

**Table V. The Relation of Fluoride Excreted to that Ingested in Water and Food**[a]

| *Ppm F in Water*[b] | *Mg F Out* | | | |
|---|---|---|---|---|
| | *Urine* | *Feces* | *Sum* | *Balance* |
| 0.1 | 0.1 | 0.05 | 0.15 | +0.05 |
| 1 | | | | |
| 2 | 2.9 | 0.4 | 3.3 | 0.3 |
| 5.5 | 4.5 | 0.6 | 5.1 | 0 |
| 6.1 | 8.1 | 0.4 | 8.5 | −0.8 |
| 8 | 10.4 | 1.4 | 11.8 | +2.0 |
| 20 | 12.3 | 1.4 | 13.7 | +8.6 |

[a] Adapted from Largent (*61*).
[b] See Table IV for total intake.

The outstanding characteristic of fluoride excretion in the urine is its speed. Sizeable fractions—for example, a quarter to a third of small doses of fluoride consumed in drinking water—are excreted in the urine of normal human adults in 3 hours. Fifty or 60% of such minute doses can be accounted for in the urine in 24 hours. Zipkin *et al.* (*107*) have shown that in individuals whose drinking water does not contain large amounts of fluoride, the urinary excretion amounts to about 0.1 mg per hour. Given a small additional dose (5 mg F), as much as 0.7 mg is excreted in the first hour, and the excretion rates thereafter decrease smoothly to reach approximately normal rates after about 10 hours. Individual variations and day-to-day variations in the urinary concentrations of fluoride are well known; *e.g.*, during a period of 10 days, one subject excreted about 0.2–0.4 mg F per day. A tea drinker with the same community water supply excreted 0.6–0.8 mg per day in the urine (*48*). The speed of fluoride excretion is most striking when the F is viewed as a possible component of the "halogen pool." Thus, the adult human body contains about 150 grams of chloride. The addition of 1.5 mg of fluoride to the circulating fluid contributes only a few parts per million to the halogen pool; nevertheless, nearly a quarter of this small amount of fluoride can be found in the urine in a period of 3 hours. Studies of the renal excretion of fluoride have shown that the rapidity can be accounted for by a somewhat less efficient tubular resorption of fluoride from the freshly formed glomerular urine than is the case with chloride. Ordinarily, 99.5% of the chloride is resorbed. For fluoride, percentage resorptions may run as low as 14–23%, although in many cases 75–94% was resorbed. Even so, the blood flow through the kidney is so large that no other explanation needs to be sought. Fluoride removal from the blood is always at a slower rate than that of creatinine, obviating the necessity of assuming that any fluoride is secreted by the kidney tubule cells.

In the relatively unexposed individual, about half of an absorbed dose of fluoride is excreted in the urine each day. The classical studies of Largent (*61*) have established this relation for doses of fluoride ranging from 1 mg to nearly 20 mg per day with an elegance seldom achieved in biological studies. In individuals ingesting small amounts of fluoride daily—*e.g.*, in a community water supply—a steady state is ultimately achieved in which the fluoride excretion almost precisely equals the fluoride intake (Tables IV and V).

When adults change water supplies, the urinary concentrations quickly approach that of the new water supply. An interesting example of the role of the skeleton in this process can be glimpsed from studies in Montgomery County following water fluoridation (*108*). In a very few weeks, the urinary fluorides of 30–39-year-old adults approached the 1 ppm concentration of the drinking water, whereas those of children, aged 5–14, gradually increased and were still only about 0.6–0.7 ppm after a year, and about 0.8 after 2 years. Most of the adult skeleton is not readily available to circulation, whereas in growing children a higher percentage of the mineral is available, and higher fractions of the ingested F are deposited, leaving less to be excreted.

Gedalia *et al.* (*32*) have recently demonstrated an interesting decrease in urinary fluoride concentration during pregnancy. Fluoride concentrations in the urine of women drinking the Jerusalem water supply (0.5–0.6 ppm F) decreased between the fourth and eighth months of pregnancy from about 0.5 ppm to nearly 0.2 ppm; the concentration rose again just before delivery. This decrease may reflect the opening of the skeleton under the influence of the normal hormones of pregnancy.

Kidney disease or injury does not seriously reduce the concentration of urinary fluoride until the kidney disease is so far advanced that signs of renal insufficiency can be observed. The urines of adult patients and children suffering from nephritis contained fluoride concentrations that did not differ significantly from those of normal individuals drinking the same water supply.

**Deposition.** Fluoride is a prototype bone seeker. In a general way, concentrations found in skeletal tissues presumably depend on the concentrations in the extracellular fluid at the time the mineral was laid down. Since the serum fluoride level has such extraordinary constancy, it is not surprising to find that neonatal bone in young animals or in human infants contains much the same concentrations of fluoride, namely 50 to 150 ppm in the ash. Fluoride deposition continues with exposure; Gedalia *et al.* (*33*) found a linear increase in the concentration of fluoride in fetal bone from the fourth month to delivery. With age, the skeletal fluoride concentration increases; the amount and the pattern of increase with long life depend on the fluoride intake. Thus, in Rochester, N. Y., before water fluoridation, the community water supply contained 0.06 ppm and the average skeletal concentrations ultimately (age 80–93 years) reached about 1200 ppm F (ash) (Figure 2). In England, Jackson and Weidmann (*52*) examined bone samples from individuals whose drinking water contained 0.5 to 2 ppm. Skeletal tissues there contained higher concentrations of fluoride and ultimately reached "steady state" at about the fiftieth to the sixtieth years of life. Bone fluoride concentrations increase linearly with increase in water fluoride levels in this country up to 4 ppm, but show less than proportionate increases at 8 ppm. Dentine and enamel also contain more fluoride with increasing concentrations of fluoride in the drinking water. Dentine usually contains approximately twice as high concentrations of fluoride as does enamel in a given locality. In a long bone, characteristic patterns of fluoride deposition are found: the concentration is lowest in the shaft and higher at each end as a result of the active growth and remodeling processes. In experimental animals, bone fluorides tend to increase in a roughly linear fashion with the logarithm of the concentration of the dietary fluoride up to a certain point. At higher levels of intake, a higher rate of increase of fluoride in the bone ash is established. The second, more rapid, phase may represent a breakdown in the homeostatic mechanisms (*3*), so that

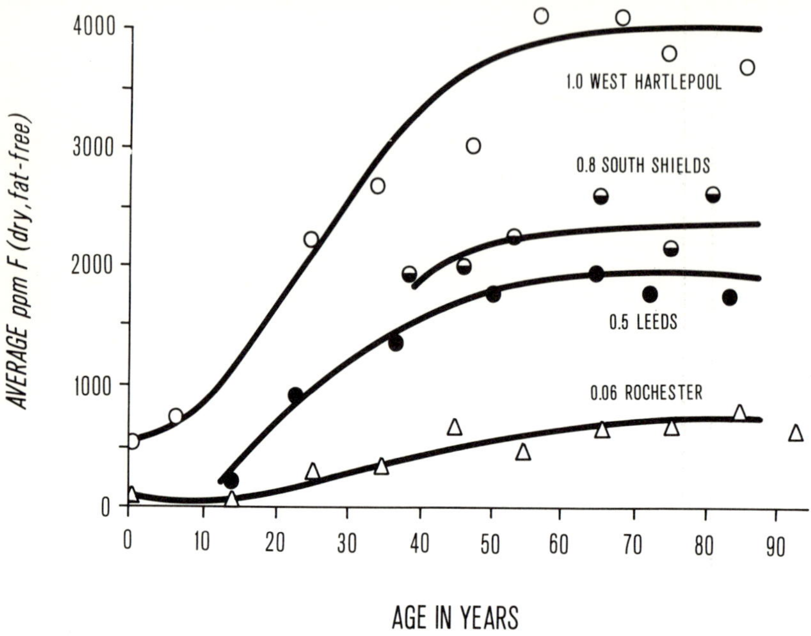


*Figure 2. Skeletal concentrations of fluoride in residents of West Hartlepool, South Shields, and Leeds, England, and Rochester, N. Y.*

the increased bone fluoride may give evidence of increased blood fluoride concentrations.

The mechanism of bone fluoride deposition from the dilute extracellular fluid (0.1 ppm) involves an exchange process in which fluoride ion replaces hydroxyl ion in the hydroxylapatite lattice to form a mixed fluorhydroxylapatite. During bone growth and mineralization, fluoride can occupy internal positions in the crystal, and the rate of fluoride deposition parallels that of phosphorus—*i.e.*, the more bone mineral formed, the more fluoride is incorporated. From concentrated fluoride solutions —*e.g.*, in topical applications of a 2% NaF solution or an 8% $SnF_2$ solution—an entirely different reaction between tooth mineral and fluoride supervenes. A layer of calcium fluoride crystals forms, and phosphate is liberated into the solution from NaF; comparable data for $SnF_2$ are not available.

Fluoride deposited in the skeleton may be mobilized either through the exchange reaction displacing fluoride from the crystal surfaces readily available to the extracellular fluids or from whole crystals dissolved by the osteoclastic–osteoblastic cycle. Largent (*61*) identified the mobilization process, which is not a simple exponential process; however, if conditions observed during the first 2 years hold, half of the skeletal fluoride would be mobilized in about 8 years.

### *Fluoride and Dental Caries*

**Water-borne Fluoride.** The public health usefulness of fluoride, specifically, its efficacy in reducing dental caries when present in optimal concentrations in community water supplies, has now been established beyond doubt (*9, 54*). First demonstrated for naturally fluoridated water by Dean and colleagues (*18*) in studies of the permanent teeth of children, the available evidence shows that the benefits persist into the adult life of individuals who continue to drink fluoridated water. Backer Dirks (*6*) recently compared caries experiences for children and adults in cities having natural or supplemented fluoridation. Adult residents of Rockford, Ill., where the water contains 0.1 ppm, have about twice as many DMF teeth at ages 20 to the 50's than were found in Aurora, Ill., where the water naturally contains 1.2 ppm F (Figure 3). The curve for adults in Rockford seems to be a fair extrapolation of the prefluoridation dental caries rates for children of various ages in Grand Rapids. After the water had been fluoridated for 10 years in Grand Rapids, the dental caries rates were notably depressed and now seem to fit reasonably

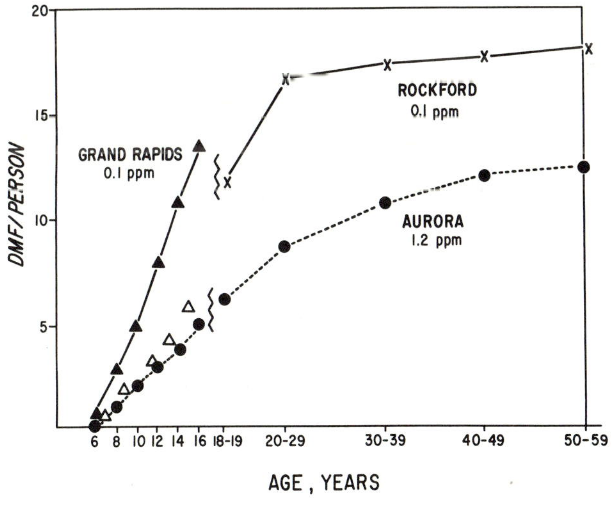


*Figure 3. Fluoride effects on dental caries*

Children: *Grand Rapids, pre-fluoridation, 0.1 ppm*—▲; *post-fluoridation, 1 ppm*—△; *Aurora, Ill., naturally, 1.2 ppm*—●. Adults: *Rockford, Ill., 0.1 ppm*—×; *Aurora, Ill., naturally, 1.2 ppm*—●

well as an extrapolation of the curve for the adult experience in Aurora. The ability of minute concentrations of fluoride to decrease dental caries is established; the optimal dose is not. "What is known? When communities (not individuals) drink fluoridated water containing 1 ppm F, the average incidence of caries (not the uniform incidence) is lowered. . . . In these communities water consumption has of course been uncontrolled and presumably highly variable. Thus, the dose of fluoride any child has consumed is not known; only on a community-wide basis is the relation between water F concentration, (and) improvement in dental health . . . known." (*44*).

**Food Fluoride.** Food fluoride has been held responsible for a unique lessening of dental caries incidence in Tristan da Cunha, where the inhabitants during periods of failure of the potato crop consumed large quantities of fish, the presumed fluoride source.

**Diet Plus Fluoride.** Food habits are difficult to alter, and, despite a considerable body of evidence pointing to dietary practices that adversely affect tooth health, dental agencies in general have had no success in obtaining public acceptance of noncariogenic human diets. In the modern U.S. community with its wealth and variety of food, water fluoridation has an appealing advantage because its beneficial action on tooth health is conferred without interfering with the food preferences of the family or of the community. During wartime, in certain countries where the amount of food was sharply curtailed with simultaneous changes in the nature of the diet, dental caries rates dropped but fluoride continued to exert a detectable effect. Weaver (*103*), for example, showed in two English communities, one with almost no fluoride in the water and the other with 1.4 ppm, that dental caries decreased in both as a result of the dietary restrictions. In 1949, both North Shields ("no F") and South Shields (1.4 ppm), consistently had fewer cavities than in 1943 (Table VI).

For many years, evidence has steadily accumulated that refined carbohydrates and particularly certain sugars in the diet increase susceptibility to tooth decay. Tank and Storvick (*97*) have shown that with increased consumption of sweets in two cities in Oregon, one (Albany) with "fluoride-free" water and the other (Corvallis) with fluoridated water (1 ppm), the caries-reducing effects of fluoride are evident both in those taking sweets frequently and in those with lesser consumption (Table VII). Tank and Storvick (*97*) have shown also the importance of breast feeding in the ultimate health of the teeth. Children who were breast fed more than 3 months have fewer cavities than those breast fed less than 3 months, who have fewer cavities than those not breast fed at all. In the same two Oregon cities, the beneficial effects of fluoride were clearly evident, superimposed on the pattern of tooth health associated with breast feeding (Table VIII).

**Table VI. Effect of Dietary Restrictions on Dental Caries in Children**[a]

| | *F, Ppm* | *No. Children, 12 Yr.* | *DMF/Child* | |
|---|---|---|---|---|
| | | | *1943* | *1949* |
| North Shields | "no F" | 500 | 4.3 | 2.4 |
| South Shields | 1.4 | 500 | 2.4 | 1.3 |

[a] From Weaver (*103*).

**Table VII. Decayed, Missing, and Filled Deciduous Teeth as Related to Frequency of Consumption of Sweets**[a]

| *Frequency Weekly Consumption Sweets* | *No. Examd.* | | *Mean Dmft*[b] | |
|---|---|---|---|---|
| | *Albany* | *Corvallis* | *Albany* | *Corvallis* |
| 0–25 | 52 | 52 | 2.7 | 2.0 |
| 26–50 | 82 | 125 | 3.6 | 1.4 |

[a] After Tank and Storvick (*97*).
[b] Dmft = decayed, missing, and filled deciduous teeth.

**Table VIII. Effect of Breast Feeding on Incidence of Decayed, Missing, and Filled Deciduous Teeth in Children One to Six Years Old**[a]

| *Extent of Breast Feeding* | *No. Examd.* | | *Mean Dmft*[b] *at 1–6 Yrs.* | |
|---|---|---|---|---|
| | *Albany* | *Corvallis* | *Albany* | *Corvallis* |
| None | 109 | 132 | 4.4 | 2.2 |
| $<$3 Mo. | 82 | 110 | 4.0 | 1.8 |
| $>$3 Mo. | 38 | 80 | 2.4 | 0.9 |

[a] After Tank and Storvick (*97*).
[b] Dmft = decayed, missing, and filled deciduous teeth.

Feltman and Kosel (*27*) have reported a fluoride tablet study in which mothers and offspring were divided into treated and control groups. An amazingly low caries incidence is reported in the treated children whose diets may have been restricted to a truly exceptional degree in "refined sugar and carbohydrate intake," coupled with presumably unusually good oral hygiene. The children, whose mothers took fluoride tablets during pregnancy, who received fluoride tablets as infants and thereafter, had no carious permanent teeth up to age 8, and averaged less than half a carious tooth per child at age 12. Unfortunately, published details of this experiment are fragmentary; confirmatory studies would have obvious interest.

Changes in dietary conditions in two cities in Japan presumably were responsible for increases in the caries rates of 12–13-year-old children during an 11-year study period. Water fluoridation at 0.6 ppm was clearly effective in maintaining a lessened incidence of caries (*71*).

Hardness of water is not a contributing factor in dental caries prevention by fluoride. Dean (*17*) found that the quantitative relation between water fluoride concentration and reduction in caries experience was independent of the total hardness of water. Surface waters are frequently lower both in fluoride and in total hardness than are deep wells; to this extent, some correlation may apparently exist. The role of certain trace elements in the incidence of dental caries and the interrelations with fluoride have been investigated recently (*10, 37*); the significance in human dental health has not been evaluated fully at present.

**Other Vehicles.** The importance of providing fluorides for those not having access to a community water supply has led to the consideration of a number of other vehicles for fluoride administration. Several have been tried or proposed—for example, fluoride solutions in the home or school (*14, 49*), fluoride for infants in vitamins or by drops, fluoride tablets or lozenges, fluoridated salt or milk, and possibly fluoride in cereal (wheat, rye, oats) or bread. Ericsson (*24*) raises a question and comments on it. "Can foodstuffs be used for controlled caries-preventive fluoride ingestion? This would mean a further step away from Nature, which taught us the fluoridation of drinking water, but human inventiveness has already found many ways of adjusting Nature to human requirements, and after all, human inventiveness is also part of nature."

**Fluoride–Vitamin Combinations.** Strean and Beaudet (*95*) in 1945 suggested the usefulness of vitamin–fluoride combinations. Several vitamin–fluoride preparations are available; more than a score are listed in *Physician's Desk Reference* 1965. Groups of 400 treated and control children, initially 2–5 years of age, were given a vitamin–F preparation for 3 years. A 63% reduction in carious permanent teeth was observed (*41, 73*).

**Fluoride Tablets.** Beginning with the report of Dietz (*19*) in 1953 on the use of fluoride tablets in caries prevention, at least a dozen subsequent papers describe studies conducted for periods up to 6 years. Most studies begin with children at 6 years of age, when they start to school. Dental caries incidence has been reduced generally 20–35% when one tablet containing 1 mg of fluoride is administered daily in school (Table IX). The maximal achievable benefit is not yet established, nor how long the protection will be exerted following the treatment period. In one study, the effectiveness of fluoride tablets was considered comparable to that of naturally or artificially fluoridated water (*5*).

**Table IX. Efficacy of Fluoride-Containing Tablets in the Reduction of Dental Caries**

| *Dose, Mg F/Day* | *No. Subjects* | *Duration, Yrs.* | *Initial Age, Yrs.* | *Reduction in Dental Caries, %* | *Reference* |
|---|---|---|---|---|---|
| 1 | — | — | — | 70 | *59* |
| 1 | >1000 | 3 | 9 | 33 | *56* |
| 1 | 21,000 | 3, 4 | 6–9 | 20–22 | *105* |
| 1 | | 4 | 6–7 | 22–26 | *64* |
| 0.5 | 1892 | 6 | 6–7 | 23 | *90* |
| 2 | 983 | 4 | 4–6 | 36 | *94* |
| 1 | | 6? | 6–7 | 29–36 | *63* |
| 1 | 296 | 6 | 6 | 19 | *40* |

**Fluoride Lozenges.** Bibby *et al.* (*7*) in 1955 reported caries reduction when fluoride lozenges were sucked, permitting the possibility of some topical action of fluoride liberated into the saliva. It is not known whether in some studies of fluoride tablets the school children let the tablets disintegrate in the mouth.

**Fluoridated Table Salt.** Fluoridated and iodized salt has been for sale in Switzerland in most of the cantons for a number of years. The World Health Organization recently initiated a fluoridated salt study in Columbia, South America. Suggested amounts of fluoride that should be added either to table salt as packaged and sold or to the salt used by bakers have ranged from 200 to 370 mg NaF/kg salt. At present in Switzerland, kitchen salt contains 200 mg NaF/kg (90 mg F/kg).

A recent report from the Wadenswil area (*66*) shows a caries reduction in the children aged 7–12 whose families used the fluoridated salt for 5 years which is similar to but about half that observed in the children of the same ages in Grand Rapids following the first 5 years of water fluoridation there. Similar results are reported from Zurich (*67*).

**Fluoridated Milk.** The caries-preventive effect of fluoride given in milk has been reported in the United States by Rusoff *et al.* (*87*) in 1962 and in Switzerland by Wirz (*104*) in 1964. In Rusoff's study, 80 school children in the age range of 6–10 years initially, for 4.5 years drank half a pint of milk daily containing 1 mg F. Control school children were given milk without fluoride. Rusoff's findings were favorable (an 80% lower incidence of dental caries); however, the groups are too small to give reliable quantitative evidence. Wirz found fluoridated milk to be approximately as effective as fluoridated water in reducing dental caries. Ericsson has shown that the fluoride in milk is available both for adsorption onto tooth surfaces and for absorption systemically (*23*).

**Fluoride in Bread.** Ericsson (*24*) reports that salt used in baking bread is being fluoridated for a test in Holland growing out of an investigation which indicated that bread is a less variable item of diet than water. Ege (*21*), in Denmark, proposes to fluoridate cereals, for example, at a level of 3.5 mg F to each kilogram. This, he believes, would also make a less variable source of fluoride than does water.

**Fluoride Dentifrices.** The effectiveness of fluorides applied in dentifrices has been repeatedly demonstrated (*46*, p. 496). The extent of the benefit is still under discussion.

**Fluoride Mouth Rinses.** Some evidence (*e.g.*, *29, 101*) of a caries-reducing effect has been presented.

The usefulness and safety of water fluoridation is buttressed by information on the tooth health and general health of the literally millions of people who have drunk naturally fluoridated water for their lifetimes, by 10-year or longer studies of adequately large groups of children in which fluoride was added to the drinking water supply, and by a great deal of animal investigation. Extensive, controlled long-range studies of each of these newer vehicles is needed before any one of them can be recommended with the same degree of confidence that water fluoridation can now be recommended.

**Mechanism.** The mechanism by which fluoride improves tooth health still remains a mystery, but some of the probable factors have been identified. A part of the protective action can be ascribed to effects on the teeth, strengthening the defense against decay, and a part to effects on oral microorganisms, dulling the edge of their disintegrative attack. Fluoride tends to alter tooth form and structure, physically and chemically, in ways that oppose dissolution; fluoride tends to reduce bacterial growth and especially bacterial acid production.

TOWARD A MORE PERFECT STRUCTURE. It was hard to accept the now established fact that fluoride, infamous 30 years ago for its grotesque disfigurement of teeth when taken in excess, is responsible at optimal levels for a more perfect structure. The number of white spots (minor imperfections of the enamel surface) are fewer when the drinking water contains 1 ppm F than at lower concentrations (*28*). About 20% of the residents of communities where only minute traces of fluoride occur in the drinking water exhibit white spots, whereas in communities with optimal fluoridation, the incidence is only 7–15%. X-ray diffraction studies reveal increasing crystallinity of bone and tooth mineral with increasing percentages of fluoride. Posner, Eanes, and colleagues (*20, 84*) have proposed that the sharpening of diffraction lines is evidence of fewer crystalline tablets (half as many in high-F bones), and of larger volume from growth in width and thickness but not along the c-axis of the hexagonal prisms. Teeth develop with more resistant forms—*e.g.*, with rounder cusps and shallower fissures.

CHEMICAL CHANGES. Changes in chemical composition occur of sorts known to be associated with lessened susceptibility to caries when water is fluoridated. The fluoride content increases especially in the most superficial layer of the enamel (Figure 4). Radiofluoride penetrates into areas of incipient caries and may confer resistance to the extension of cavities (*74*). Although the bone mineral contains less carbonate (*76, 77*) and less citrate (*109*) as the fluoride concentration increases without change in the calcium-to-phosphorus ratio, the tooth enamel carbonate is unchanged, and no relation is apparent between fluoride and citrate (*31, 69*). High carbonate concentrations are correlated with higher caries rates in experimental animals.

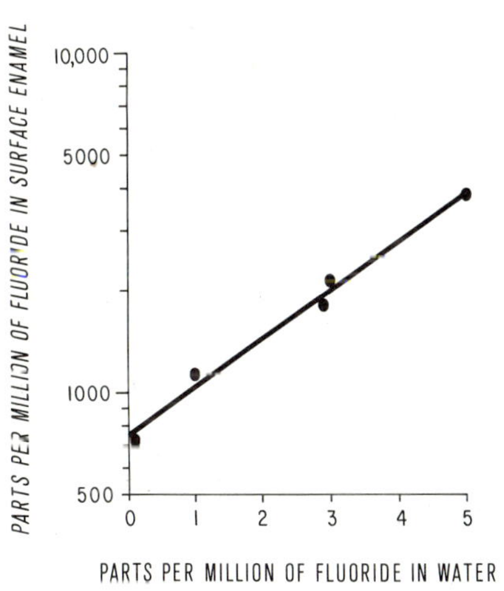


*Figure 4. Relation between water-borne fluoride and fluoride in surface enamel. Adapted from* (46)

SOLUBILITY REDUCTION. Fluoride-treated enamel dissolves in acid more slowly than untreated.

The more fluoride enamel samples naturally contain, the slower the solution rates in acid buffers (*in vitro, 51; in vivo, 57*). The solubility in body fluids of fluorapatite (and presumably of fluor-hydroxyapatite) is almost certainly less than that of hydroxyapatite.

Fluoride may facilitate nucleation and the initiation of calcification, thereby making a more highly calcified tissue.

LESSENED BACTERIAL ACID PRODUCTION. Concentrations of fluoride sufficient to reduce the rate of bacterial growth may not ordinarily occur in the mouth; however, lower and perhaps achievable concentrations decrease acid production in susceptible bacteria.

Even relatively small concentrations of fluoride—*e.g.*, 2–6 ppm—interfere with acid production in cultures of oral bacteria under certain conditions (*53, 55*).

Local F concentrations may exist near the enamel surface, available to bacteria, and effective in reducing the rate of bacterial acid production. The plaque on the surface of the teeth contains relatively high concentrations, averaging about 50 and ranging over 150 ppm F (*16, 38*). When bacteria lying in or on the plaque produce metabolic acids which diffuse toward the enamel surface mineral underneath the plaque, fluoride may be liberated, to form unionized HF at the local pH which diffuses back into the bacteria, effectively hindering further acid production.

### *Literature Cited*

(1) Abramson, E., *et al., Sv. Tandl. Tidskr.* **1954,** 47, 1.
(2) Abuladze, A. S., Pailodze, Yu. B., Kutateladze, E. A., Antelava, A. V., Glonti, L. V., *Gigiena i Sanit.* **1959,** 24, 71.
(3) Armstrong, W. D., *Arch. Oral Biol.,* **1961,** Special Suppl., 4, 156.
(4) Armstrong, W. D., Knowlton, M., *J. Dental Res.* **1942,** 21, 326.
(5) Arnold, F. A., Jr., McClure, F. J., White, C. L., *Dental Progr.* **1960,** 1, 8.
(6) Backer Dirks, O., "Advances in Fluorine Research and Dental Caries Prevention," Vol. 2, p. 33, J. L. Hardwick, J.-P. Dustin, and H. R. Held, Eds., Macmillan, New York, 1964.
(7) Bibby, B. G., Wilkins, E., Witol, E., *Oral Surg. Oral Med. Oral Pathol.* **1955,** 8, 213.
(8) Bredemann, G., "Biochemie und Physiologie des Fluors und der Industriellen Fluor-Rauchschaden," Akademie-Verlag, Berlin, 1956, 299 pp.
(9) *Brit. Dental J.* **1965,** 7, 119.
(10) Buttner, G., *J. Dental Res.* **1963,** 42 (Pt. 2), 453.
(11) Call, R. A., Greenwood, D. A., LeCheminant, W. H., Shupe, J. L., Nielsen, H. M., Olson, L. E., Lamborn, R. E., Mangelson, F. L., Davis, R. V., *Public Health Repts. (U. S.)* **1965,** 80, 529.
(12) Carlson, C. H., Armstrong, W. D., Singer, L., *Am. J. Physiol.* **1960,** 199, 187.
(13) Cholak, J., *J. Occupational Med.* **1959,** 1, 501.
(14) Council on Research, Can. Dental Assoc., *J. Can. Dental Assoc.* **1967,** 33, 506.
(15) Danielsen, M. E., Gaarder, T., *Univ. Bergen Arbok Naturvitenskap. Rekke,* **1956,** 20, 15 pp.
(16) Dawes, C., Jenkins, C. N., Hardwick, J. L., Leach, S. A., *Brit. Dental J.* **1965,** 119, 164.
(17) Dean, H. T., *J. Am. Water Works Assoc.* **1943,** 35, 1161.
(18) Dean, H. T., *Public Health Repts. (U. S.)* **1938,** 53, 1443.
(19) Dietz, V. H., *Missouri State Dental Assoc. J.* **1953,** 33, 7.
(20) Eanes, E. D., Zipkin, I., Harper, R. A., Posner, A. S., *Arch. Oral Biol.* **1965,** 10, 161.
(21) Ege, R., *Tandlaegebladet* **1961,** 65, 445.
(22) Elliott, C. G., Smith, M. D., *J. Dental Res.* **1960,** 39, 93.
(23) Ericsson, Y., *Acta Odontol. Scand.* **1958,** 16, 51.

(24) Ericsson, Y., "Effects of Fluorides in Foods," Symposia of the Swedish Nutrition Foundation, III, Gunnar Blix, Ed., Almqvist and Wiksell, Stockholm, 1965.
(25) Ericsson, Y., Malmnas, C., *Acta Obstet. Gynecol. Scand.* **1962,** 41, 144.
(26) von Fellenberg, T., *Mitt. Gebiete Lebensm. Hyg.* **1948,** 39, 124.
(27) Feltman, R., Kosel, G., *J. Dental Med.* **1961,** 16, 190.
(28) Forrest, J. R., *Brit. Dental J.* **1956,** 100, 195.
(29) Forsman, B., *Sverige Tandlakarforb Tidn* **1965,** 57, 705.
(30) Gabovich, R. D., *Gigiena i Sanit.* **1951,** 6, 31.
(31) Gedalia, I., Azaz, B., Schmerling, M., *J. Dental Res.* **1969,** 48, 105.
(32) Gedalia, I., Brzezinski, A., Bercovici, B., *J. Dental Res.* **1959,** 38, 548.
(33) Gedalia, I., Brzezinski, A., Portuguese, N., Bercovici, B., *Arch. Oral Biol.* **1964,** 9, 331.
(34) Goldman, P., *J. Biol. Chem.* **1965,** 240, 3434.
(35) Grieser, N., *Med. Ernahrung* **1965,** 6, 30.
(36) Ham, M. P., Smith, M. D., *Can. J. Res.* **1950,** 28F, 227.
(37) Hardwick, J. L., "Dental Caries and Trace Elements," Ciba Foundation Symposium, Caries-Resistant Teeth, G. E. W. Wolstenholme and M. O'Connor, Eds., Little, Brown and Co., Boston, Mass., 1965.
(38) Hardwick, J. L., Leach, S. A., "Advances in Fluorine Research and Dental Caries Prevention," J. L. Hardwick, J.-P. Dustin, and H. R. Held, Eds., Macmillan, New York, 1963.
(39) Hart, S. M., *J. Assoc. Offic. Agr. Chemists* **1961,** 44, 633.
(40) Held, A.-J., "Advances in Fluorine Research and Dental Caries Prevention," Vol. 2, p. 57, J. L. Hardwick, J.-P. Dustin, and H. R. Held, Eds., Macmillan, New York, 1964.
(41) Hennon, D. K., Stookey, G. K., Muhler, J. C., *J. Dentistry Children* **1966,** 33, 3.
(42) Heyroth, F. F., "Ingestion of Fluoride Derived from the Drinking Water and Its Elimination by Man," Progr. Rept., Public Health Service Grant **G 3363,** Dec. 1, 1951, to May 31, 1954.
(43) Hodge, H. C., "Fluoride Mineral Metabolism," Vol. II, Part A, C. L. Comar and F. Bronner, Eds., Academic Press, New York, 1964, 649 pp.
(44) Hodge, H. C., *J. Pediat.* **1963,** 63, 454.
(45) Hodge, H. C., Smith, F. A., *Ann. Rev. Pharmacol.* **1968,** 8, 395.
(46) Hodge, H. C., Smith, F. A., "Fluorine Chemistry," Vol. IV, J. H. Simons, Ed., Academic Press, New York, 1965, 786 pp.
(47) Hodge, H. C., Smith, F. A., Chen, P. S., "Fluorine Chemistry," Vol III, J. H. Simons, Ed., Academic Press, New York, 1963, 240 pp.
(48) Hodge, H. C., Smith, F. A., Gedalia, I., "Fluorides in Human Health," Y. Ericsson, Ed., World Health Organization, Geneva, in press.
(49) Horowitz, H. S., Heifetz, S. B., *Clin. Pediat.* **1966,** 5, 103.
(50) Iizuka, Y., *Nippon Eiseigaku Zasshi* **1964,** 19, 1.
(51) Isaac, S., Brudevold, F., Smith, F. A., Gardner, D. E., *J. Dental Res.* **1958,** 37, 254.
(52) Jackson, D., Weidmann, S. M., *J. Pathol. Bacteriol.* **1958,** 76, 451.
(53) Jenkins, G. N., *Arch. Oral Biol.* **1959,** 1, 33.
(54) Jenkins, G. N., *World Rev. Nutr. Dietet.* **1967,** 7, 138.
(55) Jenkins, G. N., Ferguson, D. B., Edgar, W. M., *Helv. Odontol. Acta* **1967,** 11, 2.
(56) Kessler, W., Solth, K., *Stoma* **1958,** 11, 14.
(57) King, W. J., Weiss, S., Volpe, A. R., Eigen, E., *Ann. N. Y. Acad. Sci.* **1965,** 131, 713.
(58) Kirchgessner, M., Weser, U., Friesecke, H., Oelschlager, W., *Z. Tierphysiol. Tierernahr. Futtermittelk.* **1963,** 18, 193.

(59) Knappwost, A., *Deut. Med. Wochschr.* **1956,** 81, 92.
(60) Kolomiitseva, M. G., *Vopr. Pitaniya* **1961,** 20, 55.
(61) Largent, E. J., "Fluorosis. The Health Aspects of Fluorine Compounds," Ohio State University Press, Columbus, Ohio, 1961, 186 pp.
(62) Lawrenz, M., Mitchell, H. H., *J. Nutr.* **1941,** 22, 621.
(63) Leonhardt, N., "Advances in Fluorine Research and Dental Caries Prevention," Vol. 2, p. 49, J. L. Hardwick, J.-P. Dustin, and H. R. Held, Eds., Macmillan, New York, 1964.
(64) Leonhardt, N., *Arch. Oral Biol.* **1961** (Special Suppl.), 6, 17.
(65) Longwell, J., *Roy. Soc. Promot. Health J.* **1957,** 77, 361.
(66) Marthaler, T. M., "Advances in Fluorine Research and Dental Caries Prevention," Vol. 2, p. 45, J. L. Hardwick, J.-P. Dustin, and H. R. Held, Eds., Macmillan, New York, 1964.
(67) Marthaler, T. M., *Schweiz. Monatsch. Zahn.* **1961,** 71, 671.
(68) Martin, D. J., *J. Dental Res.* **1951,** 30, 676.
(69) McCann, H. G., Brudevold, F., "Environmental Variables in Oral Disease," p. 103-118, S. J. Kreshover and F. J. McClure, Eds., Publ. 81, Am. Assoc. Advan. Sci., Washington, D. C., 1966.
(70) McClure, F. J., *Public Health Rept. (U. S.)* **1949,** 64, 1061.
(71) Minoguchi, G., *Bull. Stomatol. Kyoto Univ.* **1964,** 4, 45.
(72) Muhler, J. C., "Fluorides in Human Health," Y. Ericsson, Ed., World Health Organization, Geneva, in press.
(73) Muhler, J. C., Univ. of Indiana, Bloomington, Indiana, private communication.
(74) Myers, H. M., Hamilton, J. G., Becks, H., *J. Dental Res.* **1952,** 31, 743.
(75) Nichols, M. S., "Fluoridation as a Public Health Measure," J. H. Shaw, Ed., Am. Assoc. Advan. Sci., Washington, D. C., 1954, 232 pp.
(76) Nikiforuk, G., Grainger, R. M., "Tooth Enamel, Its Composition, Properties and Fundamental Structure," pp. 26-31, Rept. Proc. Intern. Symp., London, 1964, publ. 1965.
(77) Nikiforuk, G., McLeod, I. M., Burgess, R. C., Grainger, R. M., Brown, H. K., *J. Dental Res.* **1962,** 41, 1477.
(78) Nommik, H., "Fluorine in Swedish Agricultural Products, Soil, and Drinking Water," Esselte Aktiebolag, Stockholm, 1953, 121 pp.
(79) Oelrichs, P. B., McEwan, T., *Nature* **1961,** 190, 808.
(80) Oliveira, M. M., *Experientia* **1963,** 19, 586.
(81) Osis, D., Spencer, H., Samachson, J., *IADR Abstracts* **1969,** 148.
(82) Ostroff, J., Dept. of Health, Education, and Welfare, Public Health Service, Washington, D. C., private communication.
(83) Pisareva, M. K., *Vestnik Akad. Nauk Kazakh. SSR* **1955,** 11, 86.
(84) Posner, A. S., Eanes, E. D., Zipkin, I., Proc. Second European Symp. Calcified Tissues, pp. 79-88, Liege, Belgium, 1964.
(85) Quentin, K.-E., Souci, S. W., Indinger, J., *Z. Lebensm. Untersuch. Forsch.* **1960,** 111, 12.
(86) Reid, E., *Chinese J. Physiol.* **1936,** 10, 259.
(87) Rusoff, L. L., Konikoff, B. S., Frye, J. B., Jr., Johnston, J. E., Frye, W. W., *Am. J. Clin. Nutr.* **1962,** 11, 94.
(88) Ruzhnikova, T. N., *Vopr. Pitaniya* **1963,** 22, 86.
(89) Scassellati Sforzolini, G., Cusma, N., Mastrantonio, A., "Advances in Fluorine Research and Dental Caries Prevention," Vol. 2, p. 213, J. L. Hardwick, J.-P. Dustin, and H. R. Held, Eds., Macmillan, New York, 1964.
(90) Schutzmannsky, G., *Arch. Oral Biol.* **1961** (Special Suppl.), 6, 27.
(91) Shtifanova, A. K., *Zdravookhranenie Kazakhstana (Alma-Ata)* **1962,** 22, 60.
(92) Singer, L., Armstrong, W. D., *Arch. Oral Biol.* **1969,** 14, 1343.

(93) Smith, F. A., Gardner, D. E., University of Rochester School of Medicine and Dentistry, Rochester, N. Y., private communication.
(94) Stawinski, K., Wojciak, L., Abt, S., *Czasopismo Stomatologiczne* **1963,** 16, 611.
(95) Strean, L. P., Beaudet, J. P., *N. Y. State J. Med.* **1945,** 45, 2183.
(96) Suttie, J. W., Phillips, P. H., "Fluorine and Dental Health. The Pharmacology and Toxicology of Fluorine," J. C. Muhler and M. K. Hine, Eds., Indiana University Press, Bloomington, Ind., 1959, 216 pp.
(97) Tank, G., Storvick, C. A., *J. Am. Dental Assoc.* **1965,** 70, 394.
(98) Taves, D. R., *Nature* **1968,** 220, 582.
(99) Taves, D. R., private communication, 1969.
(100) Teply, L. J., *Food Technol.* **1958,** 12, 485.
(101) Torell, P., Ericsson, Y., *Acta Odontol. Scand.* **1965,** 23, 287.
(102) Tosteson, D. C., *Acta Physiol. Scand.* **1959,** 46, 19.
(103) Weaver, R., *Brit. Dental J.* **1950,** 88, 231.
(104) Wirz, R., *Schweiz. Monatsch. Zahn.* **1964,** 74, 767.
(105) Wrzodek, G., *Zahnartzl. Mitteil.* **1959,** 47, 258.
(106) Zimmerman, P. W., Hitchcock, A. E., Gwirtsman, J., *Contrib. Boyce Thompson Inst.* **1957,** 19, 49.
(107) Zipkin, I., Lee, W. A., Leone, N. C., *Am. J. Public Health* **1957,** 47, 848.
(108) Zipkin, I., Likins, R. C., McClure, F. J., Steere, A. C., *Public Health Repts. (U. S.)* **1956,** 71, 767.
(109) Zipkin, I., McClure, F. J., Lee, W. A., *Arch. Oral Biol.* **1960,** 2, 190.

RECEIVED August 14, 1968. Preparation of this manuscript was supported in part under contract with the U. S. Atomic Energy Commission at the University of Rochester Atomic Energy Project, Rochester, N. Y. and has been assigned report number UR-49-889 and in part by the USPHS Grant GM-15190.

# Minerals: Calcium and Phosphorus

ROBERT S. HARRIS

Massachusetts Institute of Technology, Cambridge, Mass.

*The results of over 130 studies with hamsters and rats indicate that phosphates exert a significant cariostatic action when added to caries-producing diets. Phosphates decrease in cariostatic activity depending on type of anion (cyclic-, trimeta-, tripoly-, hexameta-, ortho-, and pyro-, respectively) and type of cation (H, Na, K, Ca, and Mg, respectively). Organic phosphates (phytate, glycero-phosphate, etc.) are also effective. This cariostatic effect appears to result from a local action on the tooth as the phosphate passes through the mouth.*

Since calcium and phosphorus are the dominant constituents of teeth, it is not surprising that dental investigators have long studied the effects of deficiency of these minerals upon the development of dental caries.

The absorption of calcium from the intestine depends upon the amount of calcium ingested, the intestinal environment, and upon factors in food which may influence its uptake. High intestinal pH, extremes in the Ca/P ratios in the diet, and deficient supply of vitamin D may reduce calcium absorption. Foods rich in oxalic acid (*e.g.*, rhubarb and spinach) or in phytates (*e.g.*, unmilled cereals) may interfere with calcium absorption by forming insoluble compounds that are poorly absorbed. In spite of these factors, the human body has so great a capacity to adapt to variations in calcium intake that tooth formation is disturbed only when the deficiency is serious.

The availability of calcium and phosphorus to the tissues depends upon the activity of the parathyroid glands. Abnormal parathyroid functioning may affect the development of unerupted teeth (*31, 32*). Sobel and Hanok (*28*) have demonstrated also that the composition of the tissue fluid surrounding the developing tooth is important, and that a relationship exists between the composition of the diet, the blood, and the teeth with respect to calcium, phosphorus, and carbonate content. A deficiency of calcium in the tissue fluid may provoke a hypoplasia of the enamel which is similar to that produced by vitamin D deficiency during tooth development.

A hypoplastic line through the whole dentition has been described as resulting from a temporary disturbance in growth rate, yet the density of the calcium in this region of the tooth is essentially the same as in normal enamel. Vitamin D hypoplasia in children does not increase caries susceptibility, and an osteomalacia resulting from calcium-deficient diets does not lead to an increase in caries in pregnant women or in their offspring. Dahlberg (*5*) reported that neither calcium nor vitamin D taken during pregnancy and lactation had an influence in caries development. The evidence seems conclusive that alterations in calcium nutrition or in calcium metabolism have little effect upon dental caries development in human beings.

The effects of deficiencies and excesses of calcium and/or phosphorus upon dental caries in rats maintained on experimental diets were shown clearly in three experiments reported by the Haldi group (*7, 33, 34*). It is generally agreed that a diet containing 0.5% Ca and 0.5% P is quite adequate for rat nutrition. In Experiment A (Table I), the P content of the diet was held constant, and the Ca content was adjusted to 0.5, 1.0, 2.0, and 3.0 times its requirement. In Experiment B, the Ca content was held constant, and the P content was adjusted to 0.5, 1.0, 2.0, and 3.0 times its requirement. Finally, in Experiment C, the Ca and P contents were adjusted concurrently to 0.5, 1.0, 2.0, or 3.0 times the requirement.

**Table I. Effects of Variations in Ca and P Contents of Rat Diets upon Dental Caries Development**

| *Exp.* | *Ca/P of Diet* | *% Ca in Diet* | *% P in Diet* | *No. of Rats* | *Average No. of Lesions* | *Average Caries Score* | *Ref.* |
|---|---|---|---|---|---|---|---|
| A | 1:2.0 | 0.29 | 0.52 | 20 | 23 ± 0.4 | 34 ± 1.5 | (*7*) |
| | 1:1.0 | 0.57 | 0.50 | 20 | 21 ± 0.5 | 27 ± 1.3 | |
| | 1:0.5 | 1.01 | 0.49 | 20 | 19 ± 0.8 | 21 ± 1.2 | |
| | 1:0.3 | 1.57 | 0.52 | 20 | 17 ± 0.8 | 20 ± 1.2 | |
| B | 1:0.5 | 0.49 | 0.24 | 40 | 22 ± 4.2 | 44 ± 18 | (*34*) |
| | 1:1.0 | 0.50 | 0.52 | 40 | 18 ± 4.7 | 25 ± 11 | |
| | 1:2.0 | 0.50 | 0.98 | 40 | 13 ± 6.1 | 16 ± 8 | |
| | 1:3.0 | 0.50 | 1.48 | 40 | 11 ± 5.3 | 13 ± 8 | |
| C | 1:1 | 0.25 | 0.25 | 15 | 24 ± 2.4 | 47 ± 15 | (*33*) |
| | 1:1 | 0.50 | 0.50 | 15 | 21 ± 1.4 | 33 ± 11 | |
| | 1:1 | 1.00 | 1.00 | 15 | 18 ± 3.5 | 21 ± 6 | |
| | 1:1 | 1.50 | 1.50 | 15 | 17 ± 4.0 | 20 ± 4 | |

Deficient levels of Ca, P, or both, caused increases in caries development. The phosphorus-deficient diet was more cariogenic than the calcium-deficient diet. Excesses of either Ca, P, or both caused decreases in caries development. Excesses of P were more cariostatic than excesses of Ca and the effects on caries development were greater when the diets were deficient or excessive in both Ca and P content. It is evident that the level of dietary Ca and P was influencing caries development in rats under these special conditions.

Since phosphorus is a major component of the tooth, the diet must supply liberal amounts, especially during early growth and development. Although the diets of human beings normally contain generous amounts of phosphorus, it usually is not utilized efficiently. Much of the phosphorus in foods from plant sources (*e.g.*, cereals, legumes, leafy vegetables) is present as poorly-soluble phytates which must be degraded to orthophosphates by enzymatic hydrolysis to be utilized. Furthermore, even when phosphorus is present as orthophosphate it may react with divalent minerals (*e.g.*, Ca, Mg, Zn) in the food or in the intestinal tract to form poorly-soluble complexes. This explains why more than 50% of the phosphorus ingested in the diet generally is excreted without being absorbed.

Investigators have been slow in determining whether phosphorus plays a role in dental caries development. Possibly this has been because the Ca/P ratio of diets was being overemphasized (*11*). Lenox (*18, 19, 20*) suggested that phosphorus deficiency might be the cause of rampant caries in white populations in South Africa without presenting evidence to support the concept. This deduction resulted from an observation that the excellent teeth in native black populations resulted from consuming natural unrefined foods, while the poor teeth in white populations resulted from consuming refined foods. It has been known for some time that refined foods lose considerable minerals, including phosphates, during the milling of cereals and the refining of sugar (*24*).

Perhaps the earliest experimental evidence of a correlation between low-phosphorus diets and dental caries was presented by Klein and McCollum (*15*), who later mistakenly suggested that the particle size of the corn in the diet was responsible (*16*). Klein and Shelling (*17*), Agnew *et al.* (*1*), and Rosebury and Karshan (*25*) all observed a relationship between low dietary P and high dental caries in rats; only Shelling and Asher (*26*) failed to confirm this relationship.

Harris *et al.* (*13*) and Harris and Nizel (*10*) later observed that the ash of a mixed diet was cariostatic when added to the diet of hamsters. They analyzed this ash spectrographically and chemically, then compounded a salt mixture which duplicated the mineral elements in the food ash, and demonstrated that this salt mixture was strongly cariostatic also when added to the diet. They then modified this salt mixture by omitting one mineral element at a time. The cariostatic activity was completely lost when only phosphorus was omitted from the salt mixture. Thus, it was demonstrated that potassium orthophosphate is very effective as a cariostatic agent, even when added to a diet already nutritionally adequate in phosphorus content.

During the past decade, the results of more than 150 studies have been published by scores of scientists working in various parts of the world who supplemented various caries-producing diets by different phosphate compounds. They have been nearly unanimous in reporting that various types of inorganic and organic phosphates are effective in reducing and even preventing dental caries in rodents. Nizel and Harris (*23*) published a thorough review of this literature in 1964. The literature indicated that (a) the anticaries activities of different types of sodium phosphates decrease in the following order: trimeta-, tripoly-, hexameta-, ortho- and pyro (*14*); (b) the salts of the same anion (*e.g.*, orthophosphate) decreased in anticaries activity in the following order: $H > Na > K > Ca > Mg$; (c) organic phosphates such as Na glycerophosphate, Na phytate, or Na sucrose phosphate are equally as cariostatic as Na orthophosphate, and (d) similar relationships were found when the various phosphates were compared in rats, hamsters, or cotton rats.

McDonald *et al.* (*21*) added 1% $NaH_2PO_4$, 1% $Na_2HPO_4$, or 0.25% $NaH_2PO_4$ + 0.25% $Na_2HPO_4$ to the cariogenic diets of rats to compare the cariostatic actions of acid, alkaline, and neutral forms of sodium orthophosphate. They reported caries reductions of 61.4, 55.1, and 42.2%, respectively, after the diets had been fed for 150 days. Thus, the acid phosphate was the most active in controlling caries and the neutral phosphate mixture was the least effective. This confirmed the evidence of others (*14, 23*) that the acidity of phosphates does not interfere with their cariostatic action.

Present evidence indicates that the anticaries effects of phosphates are local, acting upon the surface layers of the teeth (*22*). A dramatic cariostatic effect was noted when the phosphate was fed immediately after tooth eruption. The mechanism of the action of phosphorus is quite different from that of fluorine. Navia and Harris (*22*) noted that phosphate delays the initiation of caries, while fluorine retards the development of caries after it has been initiated. The cariostatic actions of fluorine and phosphates are synergistic when they are fed concurrently.

Though the evidence is by no means conclusive, it appears that phosphate supplements may be effective in controlling dental caries in human beings. Six clinical studies have been conducted to date (Table II). Stralfors (*29*), Stookey *et al.* (*30*), and Harris *et al.* (*8*) added phosphates to foods, fed them to children during periods of 1 to 3 years,

**Table II. Effects of Different**

| *Test Substance* | *Level Fed: % Compound* | *Level Fed: % P* | *Vehicle* | *No. of Subjects* | *Age at Beginning: Range* | *Age at Beginning: Average* | *Test Period* |
|---|---|---|---|---|---|---|---|
| $CaHPO_4$ | 0.0<br>2.0 | <br>0.456 | Sugar & flour | 163<br>114 | 6–15<br>6–15 | –<br>– | 2<br>2 |
| $CaHPO_4 \cdot 2H_2O$ | 0.0<br>2.0 | <br>0.36 | Sugar, bread, & flour | 1001<br>1101 | 8.5–9.5<br>8.5–9.5 | 9<br>9 | 2<br>2 |
| $CaHPO_4 \cdot 2H_2O$ | 0.0<br>2.0 | <br>0.36 | Bread, cakes, & buns | 350<br>390 | 7–14<br>7–14 | 10.2<br>10.2 | 3<br>3 |
| $CaHPO_4 \cdot 2H_2O$ | 0.0<br>1.125 gm/day | <br>0.2 gm/day | Chewing gum | 129<br>138 | 6–18<br>6–18 | 12.4<br>12.4 | 2.5<br>2.5 |
| $NaH_2PO_4$[a] | 0.0<br>1.0 | <br>0.24 | Breakfast cereal | 116<br>84 | 5–16<br>5–16 | 10.1<br>10.3 | 2<br>2 |
| Ca sucrose phosphate | 0.0<br>1.0 | <br>0.062 | Flour, biscuits, syrup, & jam | 632<br>408 | 5–17<br>5–17 | –<br>– | 1<br>1 |

[a] $NaH_2PO_4$ was replaced by mixture of $NaH_2PO_4$(0.74) and $Na_2HPO_4$(0.26) at end of first year.

and noted "significant" reductions in the development of new caries, in comparison with control groups of children fed the same foods without phosphate supplementation. Finn and Jamison (*6*) noted a reduction in caries development when children chewed phosphate-enriched chewing gum daily during 2 years, in comparison with a control group that was given an identical chewing gum not fortified with phosphate. On the other hand, Averill and Bibby (*2*) and Ship and Mickelsen (*27*) failed to observe significant caries effects in somewhat similar studies in children.

The animal and clinical studies are not directly comparable. In most studies with rodents, the phosphate was incorporated into the entire diet, and was consumed concurrently whenever any food was eaten. In the clinical studies, the phosphate was added to only a portion of the food (sugar and flour; sugar, bread, and flour; bread, cakes, and buns; breakfast cereal; flour, biscuits, syrup, and jam; or in chewing gum) and not in all foods. Thus, the children in the clinical studies received less phosphate, possibly one-tenth as much, per gram of food.

**Phosphates on Dental Caries in Children**

| *DMFT* | | *DMFS* | | *DFS* | | | |
|---|---|---|---|---|---|---|---|
| *Increment per Child* | *% Reduction over Control* | *Increment per Child* | *% Reduction over Control* | *Increment per Child* | *% Reduction over Control* | *Comments* | *Ref.* |
| 5.6 | – | 9.6 | – | – | – | | (*2*) |
| 5.0 | 11 | 9.3 | 3 | | – | | |
| – | – | – | – | 0.27(m) | – | 50% & 40% reductions after 1 & 2 yrs., resp. | (*29*) |
| – | – | – | – | 0.26(f) | | | |
| | | | | 0.16(m) | 41(m) | | |
| | | | | 0.14(f) | 46(f) | | |
| 4.64 | – | 8.12 | – | – | – | | (*27*) |
| 4.43 | 4.5 | 7.41 | 9 | – | – | | |
| 3.12 | – | 5.9 | – | 5.60 | | | (*6*) |
| 2.54 | 19 | 4.7 | 20 | 4.50 | 20 | | |
| 4.49 | – | 11.45 | – | – | – | | (*30*) |
| 2.86 | 36.3[b] | 6.75 | 41.0[b] | – | – | | |
| | 16.8[b] | | 22.2[b] | | | | |
| – | – | 6.56 | – | – | – | Significant reduction in 5 to 12 yrs. age group.[c] | (*14*) |
| – | – | 5.47 | 16.6 | – | – | | |

[b] Data from two observers.
[c] Results were essentially the same at end of two years (*3*).

Dicalcium phosphate was used in four of the clinical studies, sodium orthophosphate was used in the fifth, and calcium sucrose phosphate was used in the sixth. Harris *et al.* (*8, 9, 14*) and Cagnone *et al.* (*4*) demonstrated in rats that sodium trimetaphosphate is approximately five times as effective as a cariostatic agent as sodium orthophosphate, and Harris and Nizel (*12*) have shown that phosphorus in the form of sodium orthophosphate is possibly three times more effective than phosphorus in calcium orthophosphate. Phosphate in calcium sucrose phosphate is less effective than phosphate in sodium orthophosphate. Sodium trimetaphosphate is the most effective of all phosphates yet tested in animals, is less toxic than orthophosphate, and appears to be the compound of choice for clinical trials.

Calcium and phosphorus can influence the development of caries when added to the diet, to chewing gum, or to other carriers; phosphate is more effective than calcium as a cariostatic agent, and both calcium and phosphate are effective even when added as supplements to diets already nutritionally adequate.

### *Literature Cited*


(1) Agnew, M. C., Agnew, R. S., Tisdall, F. F., *J. Am. Dental Assoc.* **1933,** 20, 193.
(2) Averill, H. M., Bibby, B. G., *J. Dental Res.* **1964,** 43, 1150.
(3) Beveridge, J., Gregory, G., Schamschule, R. G., Savage, D. C. L., *Med. J. Australia* **1968**, 2, 256.
(4) Cagnone, L. D., Harris, R. S., Navia, J. M., *Proc. Intern. Assoc. Dental Res.* **1968,** Abst. 364, p. 128.
(5) Dahlberg, B., *Acta Genet. Statist. Med. (Basel)* **1951,** II, 57.
(6) Finn, S. B., Jamison, H. C., *J. Am. Dental Assoc.* **1967,** 74, 987.
(7) Haldi, J., Wynn, W., Bentley, K. D., Law, M. L., *J. Nutr.* **1959,** 67, 645.
(8) Harris, R., Schamschula, R. G., Gregory, G., Roots, M., Beveridge, J., *Australian Dental J.* **1967**, 12, 105.
(9) Harris, R. S., Das, S. K., Nizel, A. E., *J. Dental Res.* **1965,** 44, 549.
(10) Harris, R. S., Nizel, A. E., *J. Dental Res.* **1959,** 38, 1142.
(11) *Ibid.,* **1964,** 43, 1090.
(12) *Ibid.,* **1965,** 44, 416.
(13) Harris, R. S., Nizel, A. E., Gardner, D. S., *Proc. Intern. Nutr. Congr., 4th,* **1957,** p. 195.
(14) Harris, R. S., Nizel, A. E., Walsh, N. B., *J. Dental Res.* **1967,** 46, 290.
(15) Klein, H., McCollum, E. V., *Science* **1931,** 74, 662.
(16) Klein, H., McCollum, E. V., *J. Dental Res.* **1932,** 13, 69.
(17) Klein, H., Shelling, D. H., *J. Dental Res.* **1931**, 11, 458.
(18) Lennox, J., *S. African Dental J.* **1929,** 3, 125.
(19) *Ibid.,* **1930,** 4, 592.
(20) *Ibid.,* **1931,** 5, 156.
(21) McDonald, J. L., Stookey, G. K., Muhler, J. C., *Arch. Oral Biol.* **1968,** 13, 903.
(22) Navia, J. M., Lopez, H., Harris, R. S., *Arch. Oral Biol.* **1968,** 13, 779.
(23) Nizel, A. E., Harris, R. S., *J. Dental Res.* **1964,** 43, 1123.
(24) Roos, A., "Kulturzerfall und Zahnverderbnis," Hans Huber, Bern, 1963.
(25) Rosebury, T., Karshan, M., *Arch. Pathol.* **1935**, 20, 697.
(26) Shelling, D. H., Asher, D. E., *J. Dental Res.* **1933,** 13, 363.
(27) Ship, I. I., Mickelsen, O. J., *J. Dental Res.* **1964,** 43, 1144.
(28) Sobel, A. E., Hanok, A., *J. Biol. Chem.* **1948,** 176, 1103.
(29) Stralfors, A., *J. Dental Res.* **1964,** 43, 1137.
(30) Stookey, G. K., Carroll, R. A., Muhler, J. C., *J. Am. Dental Assoc.* **1967,** 74, 752.
(31) Widdowson, E. M., *Voeding, Neth. J. Nutr.* **1962,** 23, 62.
(32) Wynn, W., *J. Nutr.* **1959,** 67, 645.
(33) Wynn, W., Haldi, J., Bentley, K. D., Law, M. L., *J. Dental Res.* **1960,** 39, 1248.
(34) Wynn, W., Haldi, J., Bentley, K. D., Law, M. L., *J. Nutr.* **1956,** 58, 325.


RECEIVED October 27, 1969.

# 9

# Effect of Minerals on Dental Caries

JUAN M. NAVIA[1]

Massachusetts Institute of Technology, Cambridge, Mass.

*Minerals in foods and drinking water have an important role in dental caries. Trace elements can be incorporated preeruptively and posteruptively into tooth enamel and change its physicochemical properties, affect the remineralization processes on the enamel surface, and influence the implantation and metabolism of cariogenic microorganism. Some elements promote caries, such as Se, Mg, and Cd, while others, such as Mo, V, and Sr, are mildly cariostatic. The effect of many other elements on caries is not known clearly owing to experimental limitations of the animal models used to study them. The species of animals used, the type of oral flora, the toxicity effects, and the interrelations between elements have to be evaluated and defined before a clear understanding of the role of trace elements in human caries is achieved.*

The concept that nutritional deficiencies are related to infection has been documented amply in the literature (*166*). Attempts to show through epidemiological studies that optimum nutrition inhibits dental caries, an infectious oral disease, have been unsuccessful (*157*). Caries prevalence is markedly lower in more isolated or primitive areas where the nutritional status is definitely poorer than in sections of the country with access to technical developments characteristic of modern civilization (*156*).

This observation was voiced 30 years ago when Brekhus and Armstrong (*21*) stated that dental caries is a disease of civilization and that freedom from caries, found in societies less technically advanced, results from other factors besides nutrition. Dental decay is increasing among

[1] Present address: Institute of Dental Research, University of Alabama in Birmingham, Birmingham, Ala. 35233.

technically developing nations and is rapidly approaching the severity levels found in affluent societies. A report by Baume (*12*) describes the dental and nutritional status of the school population of French Polynesia and illustrates the point. The worst dental conditions of the entire territory were found in the developing district of Papeete. Among the indigenous pre-school children, an odontoclastic type of rampant caries prevailed, particularly among those of Chinese extraction. Almost immediately after eruption of "yellow" permanent teeth, a smooth-surface type of caries "melted down" these hypoplastic teeth so that at age 13 to 15 years the Tahitians are practically edentulous.

The teeth of youngsters raised on a deficient diet are not able to withstand the impact of the caries-promoting diet consumed in urban locations while the inhabitants of distant islands, who still adhere to their traditional food habits, maintain good dental health. The change in dietary habits associated with technical and economic development probably is responsible for this deterioration in dental health which may bring rampant disease to some population groups within a generation.

One factor that has interfered with efforts to understand the nature and extent of the interaction between nutrition and dental caries is the diverse effect of nutrients (and nonnutrients) in the diet during the pre-eruptive and post-eruptive periods of tooth development. Pre-eruptively, nutrients in the diet can influence the maturation process, the chemical composition of teeth, tooth size and morphology and, to a lesser extent, the time of eruption. Nutrients in the diet also can select out the cariogenic flora by the process of enrichment and thus facilitate the implantation and colonization of these microorganisms on the tooth surface once it has erupted into the oral environment. Post-eruptively, diet can influence plaque formation and the microbial metabolic activity in the micro-environment of teeth, the composition of saliva bathing the teeth, and the composition of the enamel surface. The pre-eruptive and post-eruptive effects of diet on the development and maintenance of teeth have not always been clearly separted in experimental designs and have confused the interpretation of some results.

While most nutrients may have their major effect on dental structures pre-eruptively during the process of growth and development, minerals have a profound influence pre-eruptively and post-eruptively and, therefore, play a major role in the caries susceptibility or resistance of the tooth. The inorganic portion of protective foods will contribute practically all of the caries-protective action of the food (*14*).

From the standpoint of nutrition, mineral elements are either essential for the maintenance of life processes or nonessential. Because of their ubiquitousness, they may enter the tissues in an adventitious manner when present in the food and water consumed or in the air inhaled.

The minerals present in animal tissues can be arbitrarily divided into major elements or macrominerals, such as Ca, P, Mg, Na, K, S, and Cl, and trace elements or microminerals, such as Cu, Co, Fe, I, Mn, Mo, Se, and Zn, which are known today as the eight essential elements. Another group of trace elements which includes Al, As, B, Ba, Be, F, Hg, Ni, Rb, Si, Sr, and V may be present, but as yet no specific function has been attached to them. Some elements such as V and Sr possibly may be shown essential in future investigations.

The major mineral elements in the animal body are deposited in bone and teeth, where they either increase the rigidity of bones or serve as storage for use by tissue cells when necessary in order to maintain the integrity of metabolic functions. Trace elements may enter enzyme reactions as activators which bring the enzyme into a catalytically active state. Enzyme activity is affected by the presence or absence of mineral salts, the nature of the ions present, and their concentrations. Certain elements such as Zn, Cu, and Mo are essential structural components of enzymes such as carbonic anhydrase, polyphenol oxidase, and xanthine oxidase, respectively, while others like Ag, Hg, and Pb may be highly inhibitory to enzymes.

The requirements of animal organisms for trace elements is unknown to a large extent. They are present in tissues at extremely low concentrations, and because in their metabolic activity they are recycled and poorly excreted, their re-utilization by the tissues is nearly complete. Examples of these cycles are the metabolic re-utilization of iron and iodine.

Only in periods of nutritional stress or increased metabolic activity such as growth and development, pregnancy, or lactation is the requirement of these elements increased. Even in these circumstances, the biological reserves in organs such as the liver or bones usually are sufficient to offset a nutritional deficiency.

The whole subject of trace element requirements is in great need of a serious, dedicated experimental study.

The theory that the mineral portions of foods can affect dental caries has been substantiated by "natural" geographic experiments where a high or low incidence of caries in humans appears to be associated with a deficiency or excess of a certain element in the soil and plants grown in a locality and animal caries experiments.

**Geographic Variations in Caries and Trace Elements.** Adler and coworkers (*2*, *3*) have reported on the influence of molybdenum on dental caries in Hungary. They showed that in areas where the Mo level in the water was 0.1 ppm there was a low incidence of caries.

In 1955, Hewat and Eastcott (*85*) suggested that a possible correlation exists between caries incidence and soil composition in New Zealand. In order to study this subject further, Ludwig *et al.* (*107*) compared the caries incidence of two populations of children in two adjacent cities (Napier and Hastings). They found that the Napier children had considerably less caries than the Hastings children of comparable age (5–8 years). The results of later studies (*108*) indicated that molybdenum might be involved, and the lower caries experience of Napier children was the result of a higher Mo availability from the soil which caused increases in the mineral composition of vegetables consumed in the area. Recently, Anderson (*5, 6*) reported first a study with 270 children and then another study with larger numbers of children from the Somerset area in England. This region is one in which cattle suffer from molybdenum poisoning. When the DMF from the children in the control areas was compared with the DMF from children in the high Mo areas, it was found that the latter had better than a 20% reduction in DMF.

Other epidemiological studies have suggested that high levels of certain elements such as selenium in the soil may be associated with high caries incidence (*68*).

In this country, Nizel and Bibby (*141*) demonstrated correlations between soils and caries prevalence. The highest prevalence of caries in the United States is found in the New England states associated with podzols. These soils are generally strongly acid and of natural fertility. The lowest incidence of caries is found in the southwestern states where the semi-acid soils are potentially high in mineral nutrients for they have not been exposed to the leaching and erosion action for long periods of time. Fluoride in these soils definitely contributes to this low caries prevalence, but in the Dakotas where water high in fluoride is common, there is a fairly high prevalence of caries. This indicates that factors other than fluoride are influencing the caries picture.

**Dietary Minerals, Food Ashes, and Experimental Dental Caries.** Minerals in diets have a profound effect on the dental caries experience of experimental animals.

Sognnaes and Shaw (*172, 173*) observed more caries lesions when rats were given a purified ration that was complete in known essentials than when this ration was supplemented with 2% of its own ash. They suggested that protection against caries resulted from certain trace elements in the ash. In the light of what is known today about the cariostatic effect of phosphate, this also could be explained as arising from the P content of the ash. Keyes (*96*) observed an increase in caries activity when hamsters were fed a mineral-deficient diet. A similar effect was reported by Gustafson (*64*) who noted a marked increase in caries development when the amount of salt mixture in the diet was decreased.

The ashes of different foods decrease the incidence of caries: corn (*75*), bone (*8, 84*), and cocoa (*97, 155*). Cocoa ash has been reported inactive as a cariostatic agent by Wynn *et al.* (*214*), but Stralfors (*183,*

*184, 185*) found activity in the whole defatted cocoa. Phenolic compounds (*186*) present in cocoa might be involved in this effect. Of these foods, corn is the most important since it is commonly eaten by mankind. In 1950 (*142*), Nizel and Harris reported that diets containing corn and milk grown in Texas caused only 40% as much dental decay in hamsters as corn and milk grown in New England. This effect was not caused by fluorine since the F content was made equal by the addition of sodium fluoride to the New England diet. Later, these investigators reported (*144*) that these differences indicate the presence of a cariogenic factor in the New England corn and milk rather than the presence of a cariostatic factor in the Texas corn and milk. Reasoning that the cariogenic factor in New England foods was a trace element, Nizel and Harris (*143*) tried to magnify the effect by supplementing the New England diet with its ash (550°C). Contrary to expectations, the caries score of the hamsters fed the ash-supplemented diet was only 35% as high as the control group.

This observation led to an investigation to identify the cariostatic factor in the food ash. The composition of this ash was determined by chemical and spectrographic methods, and a salt was prepared duplicating the 11 mineral elements that could be quantitated. When fed to hamsters, this salt mixture was significantly more cariostatic than the ash which it imitated (*75*). This result could indicate that one (or more) of the trace elements in the food ash which could not be quantitated and was, therefore, omitted from the salt mixture, is a strong cariogenic agent.

In order to investigate this phenomenon further, Harris and Nizel (*74*) fed hamsters five diets containing different combinations of the 11 elements supplemented to a caries-promoting diet.

When the phosphorus component ($KH_2PO_4$) was omitted, the caries score rose from 0.7 to 18.4. Since the score of the control group was 13.4, it was evident that some of the 10 mineral elements in the P-free salt mixture might be actually cariogenic.

Constant *et al.* (*42*) carried out studies comparing whole cereals with processed and purified cereals. They found that whole cereals were less cariogenic than the purified processed product. They also investigated the cariogenicity of alkaline ash foods and that of acid ash foods and found no significant difference under the experimental conditions used. Later, they studied (*43, 44*) the effect on caries of acidic and basic minerals and found that acidic inorganic, basic, or acidic organic salt mixtures gave no protection against tooth decay, while a high level of basic inorganic salts resulted in a marked decrease in tooth decay.

Miller (*118*) reported that doubling the Hubbell-Mendel-Wakeman salt mixture from 1.2 grams to 2.4 grams/100 grams gave a marked reduction in the number of carious teeth, the number of carious areas, and the caries score. This effect was verified again in a second experiment but the effect was nullified when 12% of powdered sucrose was used in place of an equal amount of rice flour.

Even though there is a definite relation between dietary trace elements and dental caries, there is no certain knowledge of the mechanism through which these elements influence caries. Some of the possible ways in which they could act are the following:

(1) Incorporating trace elements pre-eruptively into the tooth mineral to change its physico-chemical properties.
(2) Influencing the cellular enzyme systems involved in the mineralization of the teeth.
(3) Altering pre-eruptively the nature of the calcifying organic matrix of the tooth.
(4) Enhancing or inhibiting the deposition of mineral elements such as fluoride or phosphorus on the enamel surface and thereby influencing the post-eruptive maturation of hypomineralized enamel areas.
(5) Changing the physical and chemical characteristics of saliva.
(6) Interfering directly with the reproduction, metabolism, and implantation of the cariogenic microorganisms on the tooth surface.

**Metal Ions as Enzyme Activators in Microbial Cells.** Metals may enter enzyme reactions as cofactors or activators which bring the enzyme into a catalytically active state. The activity of enzymes is affected by the presence or absence of mineral salts, the nature of the ions present, and their concentrations. Certain ions are necessary for the activity of the enzyme, while others—*i.e.*, $Ag^{+}$, $Hg^{2+}$, $Pb^{2+}$—may be highly toxic. It is a characteristic of these systems that certain ions are poisonous for some enzymes and activators for others. Some may inhibit an enzyme at one concentration and yet activate the same enzyme at another concentration. The effects of metals on enzymes may be produced by many metabolic routes, and in most cases have not been identified.

The activating effect usually is not specific. The enzyme fumarase may be activated by several metal ions, yet other enzymes such as inorganic pyrophosphatase specifically require $Mg^{2+}$ which cannot be replaced by others.

Approximately 16 different metal cations activate one or more enzymes; these are:

| | | | |
|---|---|---|---|
| $Al^{3+}$ | $Cr^{3+}$ | $K^{+}$ | $Na^{+}$ |
| $Ca^{2+}$ | $Cs^{+}$ | $Mg^{2+}$ | $Ni^{2+}$ |
| $Cd^{2+}$ | $Cu^{2+}$ | $Mn^{2+}$ | $Rb^{+}$ |
| $Co^{2+}$ | $Fe^{2+}$ | $Mo^{+}$ | $Zn^{2+}$ |

$Mg^{2+}$ is the natural activator of a great majority of the enzymes which act on phosphorylated substrates, such as the phosphokinases, the synthetases, and the enzymes which hydrolyze phosphoric acid anhydrides, but not the phosphorylases. In most cases, $Mg^{2+}$ can be replaced by $Mn^{2+}$ but not by other metals. Sodium can be replaced by $K^{+}$ in some cases, and $Mn^{2+}$, $Co^{2+}$, $Ni^{2+}$, and $Zn^{2+}$ many times are interchangeable among them. Antagonism is fairly common, and $Na^{+}$ may act as a competitive inhibitor for $K^{+}$ activation (*i.e.*, phosphotransacetylase), $Ca^{2+}$ competes with $Mg^{2+}$ to inhibit certain enzymes, such as adenosinetriphosphatase, and also $Mg^{2+}$ inhibits the $Ca^{2+}$ activation of myosin adenosinetriphosphatase. Enzymes also may be affected considerably by the presence of certain anions. Salivary alpha amylases, for example, are affected so greatly by chlorides that this ion has been regarded as the natural activator of these enzymes (*129*).

MacDonald (*116*) has discussed the microbiology of caries, stressing that it is a bacterially-induced disease characterized by a decalcifying action on the mineral components and a proteolytic action on the organic components. Given energy and nitrogen sources, the oral microbiota, in common with all microorganisms, will not grow in the complete absence of certain mineral elements. As discussed above, this is because of the role of metals as ion activators of the enzyme systems essential for metabolic activity. It would be of interest to determine the specific nutritional needs for trace elements of the cariogenic streptococci and compare them with those of the noncariogenic streptococci. Bowen (*17*) attempted to obtain such information and reported that of the three cations tested (manganese, calcium, and magnesium) only manganese is an essential requirement for growth. Although no qualitative differences were observed concerning the requirements for growth of cariogenic and noncariogenic organisms, some discrepancies in their quantitative needs were reported which warrant further research.

The minerals found in the surface enamel and those supplied by the diet, the saliva, and desquamented tissue cells may influence the oral microbiota in the following ways: stimulation of growth (increase in cell numbers), facilitation of attachment of cells to enamel surface, influencing the formation of metabolic end products including intra- and extracellular polysaccharides, inhibition of growth or metabolic activity through poisoning of enzyme systems within the cells, and modification of oral environment by stimulation of growth of certain types of cells, thus inhibiting others.

### *Mineral Composition of Teeth in Humans and Experimental Animals*

**Inorganic Composition of Bones and Teeth.** Bone and tooth mineral is made up mostly of calcium and phosphate in the form of apatite, yet many other elements are found within its structure. Bone and tooth mineral, therefore, is not a single homogeneous chemical compound but a mixture which varies in composition and distribution.

One of the problems in defining the chemical behavior of the inorganic portion of the teeth is the difficulty in differentiating between the constituents of the basic structure, the ions having only a surface relationship to the crystals, and those possibly combined with the apatite crystals in a separate phase. Therefore, even though the structure and composition of the mineral corresponds closely to that of hydroxyapatite, substantial amounts of carbonate and citrate are found as well as ion substitutions in the crystal lattice.

The minute crystals and interspaces between them expose a large surface area to the environment fluids and as a result dissolution and recrystallization may take place, maintaining a dynamic balance. This large surface area of bone and tooth minerals influences its total composition in two ways, by adsorbing or substituting ions as well as incorporating some of them within surface unit cells with unshared sides and by isoionic or heteroionic exchange with the fluids bathing the crystals.

In general, the elements which localize in bone and teeth are referred to as "bone-seekers" but the term should apply also to other organic substances such as murexide and the tetracyclines which combine avidly with bone or tooth at new calcification and also at carious sites.

**Table I. Composition of Outer and Inner Enamel of Teeth from Human Subjects Living in Different Geographic Areas**[a]

| | *µMol. per Gram* | |
|---|---|---|
| | *Outer Enamel* | *Body Enamel* |
| Carbonate | 350–440 | 525–654 |
| Sodium | 230–360 | 310–380 |
| Fluoride | 17–176 | 3.8–44 |
| Magnesium | 30–60 | 60–74 |
| Zinc | 6.6–27.5 | 2.9–14.2 |
| Citrate | 3.5–5.0 | –1.1 |
| Aluminum | 1.4–4.8 | 1.1–4.5 |
| Strontium | 0.3–3.7 | 0.7–4.6 |
| Lactate | –2.9 | –1.2 |
| Lead | 0.4–2.6 | 0.1–1.1 |
| Copper | 0.1–1.8 | tr–0.6 |
| Silica | 0.2–1.5 | 0.1–1.8 |
| Silver | tr–0.9 | 0.0–0.5 |
| Iron | 0.4–0.6 | 0.2–0.4 |
| Tin | tr–0.4 | 0.0–0.3 |
| Manganese | 0.1–0.4 | 0.1–0.2 |

[a] Data from Ref. *24*.

**Table II. Major Inorganic Constituents of Human Enamel**[a]

| *Constituent* | *Thermal Neutron Activation Analysis* | *Chemical Analysis* |
|---|---|---|
| Ca | 37.4 ± 1.0 | 33.6–39.4 |
| P | 18.3 ± 2.2 | 16.1–18.0 |
| Ca/P | 2.04 | 1.92–2.17 |
| $CO_2$ | – | 1.95–3.66 |
| Na | 1.16 ± 0.40 | 0.25–0.90 |
| Mg | 0.36 ± 0.04 | 0.25–0.56 |
| Cl | 0.65 ± 0.30 | 0.19–0.30 |
| K | – | 0.05–0.30 |

[a] Data from Ref. *175* and *176*.

**Table III. Minor Inorganic Constituents of Human Enamel**[a]

| *Constituent* | *Thermal Neutron Activation Analysis* | *Chemical Analysis* |
|---|---|---|
| F | | 62–650 |
| Fe | 388 ± 109 | 8–218 |
| Zn | 276 + 106 | 152–227 |
| Sr | 94 ± 22 | 50–400 |
| Rb | 4.9 ± 1.6 | – |
| Br | 4.6 ± 1.1 | – |
| W | 0.24 ± 0.12 | – |
| Cu | 0.26 ± 0.11 | 10–100 |
| Mn | 0.51 ± 0.08 | 0–18 |
| Au | 0.02 + 0.01 | – |
| Ag | 0.0049 ± 0.0012 | 0–100 |
| Cr | 0.0027 ± 0.0016 | – |
| Co | 0.00024 ± 0.00009 | – |
| V | $>10^{-5}$ | – |
| Pt | $>10^{-6}$ | – |

[a] Parts per million, dry weight; data from Ref. *175* and *176*.

The chemical composition of enamel, dentin, cementum, and pulp has been discussed by Zipkin (*217*), who also discussed the chemistry of the sound and carious enamel.

Brudevold (*24, 30*) reported on the trace mineral content of teeth collected from human beings living in different geographic areas. The concentrations of these elements ($\mu$M/gram) of the surface enamel and the body of the intact enamel are presented in Table I. The amounts in the outer enamel were often, but not always, higher than amounts in the inner enamel, and the range of values is quite wide. Soremark and co-workers (*175, 176*), using neutron activation analysis, reported values for total human enamel (Tables II, III).

Steadman *et al.* (*179*) analyzed the ancient teeth of Pueblo Indians (800 years old) and Indian Knoll (5000 years old) for the same elements and found that they occurred in greater concentration in the outer than in the inner layers of enamel. Fluoride was found in greatest concentration in the external enamel, followed by Zn, Si, Mn, Pb, Ag, Cu, and Sn. They noted a remarkable similarity in the distribution of many trace elements between ancient and contemporary American teeth. Contrary to expectations, they found but little penetration of trace elements into the bulk of the tooth structure, even in teeth of 5000 years old. Asgar (*7*) studied differences in the dentin and enamel of ancient Greek and American teeth, but his samples were too few to permit conclusions.

Hadjimarkos and Bonhorst (*69*) studied 27 sound and 17 carious teeth from 20–40 year old modern Athenians, and 14 sound teeth from the skulls of five women and four men who lived in 800 and 1100 B.C. (Table IV). He attributed the high immunity to caries of Athens school children to the high intake of fluoride and possibly the lower intake of selenium.

**Table IV. Mineral Content of Greek Teeth**

| | *Modern Greek* | | *Ancient Greek* | |
|---|---|---|---|---|
| | *Enamel* | *Dentine* | *Enamel* | *Dentine* |
| Fluorine, ppm | 178 | | 374 | |
| Selenium, ppm | 0.03 | 0.13 | 0.13 | 0.45 |

Several attempts have been made to correlate variations in the mineral content of dental tissues with caries sensitivity. Picard *et al.* (*148*) divided 120 human teeth into three groups: healthy, superficial caries, and deep caries. They found no significant difference in the ash, Ca, and P content, or in the Ca/P ratio of the enamel of the three groups. The ash, Ca, and P content of the dentin from deep carious lesions were significantly lower than in the healthy teeth. The same trend was noted in the teeth with superficial caries, but the trend was not significant. Lobene (*105*) studied the inorganic constituents of the enamel and dentin of teeth from hamsters, and concluded that the Ca, P, and Mg content of the dentin did not vary greatly, whatever the source.

Zipkin and Piez (*218*) tried to correlate the citric acid content of human teeth with susceptibility to caries in a study of 65 samples of sound dentin and 129 samples of carious dentin. They found 888 ± 103 mg % and 872 ± 105 mg % citric acid in the sound and carious dentin, respectively, and thus no evidence of a correlation between citric acid and dental caries. Studies of this type are difficult to interpret, for the analysis is made on the carious material left after the disease has progressed and no information is available as to the concentration of minerals before the carious lesion started.

**Trace Element Distribution in Teeth.** The distribution of individual elements in human teeth has been studied by Brudevold (*24*) and his associates. The range of copper (*47*) in four successive grindings of the enamel of human teeth was 15 to 30 ppm, and its distribution was random and unaffected by age. The tin content of pooled samples (*28*) of four successive layers of enamel was 7.0 ppm in the outer two layers and nil in the third and fourth layers. Lead (*27*) was highest (550 ppm) in the outer enamel layers of erupted teeth and decreased to a rather constant level (90 ppm) in the innermost layers. Zinc (*31*) was distributed like lead and fluoride. It was higher on the surface (430–2100 ppm), lower in the subsurface layers, and was deposited irregularly on the surface.

Little and Brudevold (*104*) found differences in the $CO_2$ content of the superficial and inner layers of intact human enamel in erupted and unerupted teeth. In all age groups, the concentration of carbon dioxide increased from the surface toward the dentin, but as the calcification proceeds during development, the carbon dioxide content decreases.

Bone-seeking radioactive isotopes (*i.e.*, Sr) accumulate in teeth. Holgate *et al.* (*87*) studied the accumulation of $Sr^{90}$ in the dental tissues of rabbits. An increase in concentration was observed during 30 days following intravenous injection, and then it fell abruptly. Since the teeth of the rabbit grow continuously, the $Sr^{90}$ deposited in the teeth may have been lost when the radioactive zone was worn away. Butler (*33*) observed an inverse correlation between the concentration of $Sr^{90}$ and the age of human beings.

The mineral composition of teeth has been studied in relation to discoloration of the tooth substance. Isaac and Brudevold (*89*) studied the possible staining properties of Pb, Sn, Ag, Hg, Cu, and Fe when deposited in the enamel, and then exposed them to a sulfur-containing medium. These metal sulfides are brown or black, and they may be produced from food or saliva under ordinary conditions. The surfaces of the crowns and roots of intact teeth were treated with solutions containing the cations, and all developed discoloration when exposed to the sulfur-containing medium. On the other hand, Landing *et al.* (*101*) noted that the teeth of a patient with hemosiderosis were not pigmented, even though they contained 50.8 $\mu$g % of iron rather than the 16.1 $\mu$g % in control patients. It is not known whether the Fe was deposited in the teeth before or after eruption. Possibly, the location of the Fe in the tooth determines whether it will be reactive.

During the last 10 years, investigators have been making use of analytical procedures based on physical principles to quantitate elements in teeth and bones. Using neutron activation analysis, Soremark and coworkers (*109, 174, 175, 176*) studied the enamel composition of normal human erupted and unerupted enamel. Nixon *et al.* (*138, 139, 140*) studied the copper, arsenic, and antimony levels in human enamel. Manganese also has been estimated in human enamel by these same investigators (*137*) and by Battistone *et al.* (*11*).

The inorganic components of teeth also have been analyzed by such methods as x-ray emission spectrography (*38*) and spark source mass spectrography (*188*). This last method continues to play an extremely important role in elemental and trace analysis because of great sensitivity for metals and nonmetals.

In general, these methods have been useful in detecting and quantitating trace quantities of elements in teeth and bone, but the development of the electron probe made possible the determination of the distribution of elements in microstructures. Equipment to produce beams of ions, protons, electrons, and x-rays is now available to be used in exploring the crystalline nature of solids and biological tissues. The electron probe has been used in metallurgy and minerology, but its applicability to biological samples has been limited by the fact that light elements which are of great interest to the biologist have not been detected easily and the physical properties of biological specimens are different from those samples normally studied in metallurgy. Today, new improvements in equipment and methodology are making possible the application of this valuable analytical tool to samples of biological origin (*4, 197, 198*).

The mineralized tissues of the body, such as bones and teeth, lend themselves to study by the probe. A narrow beam of electrons is focused on a small area of the sample (less than 1 micron in diameter), and the x-rays resulting from the electron bombardment are collected at a predetermined angle and analyzed in one or more spectrometers. These analyses can be made quantitative by comparing the counts per minute obtained with those from suitable standards. Birks (*16*) described the instrument and its use in a variety of analytical applications. Campbell and Brown (*39*) reviewed the significant progress made in the last few years.

Using the electron probe, Rosser *et al.* (*154*) studied the Ca concentration in developing enamel, and Boyde, Switsur, and Fearnhead (*19*) studied the calcium and iron distribution in rat enamel and human molar enamel. These investigators reported a higher concentration of calcium in the peritubular area of dentin than in the intertubular area. Takuma *et al.* (*189*), using an electron microscope with an x-ray spectrometer attachment, examined horse dentin prepared for routine electron microscopy (500 A thick). They found twice as much Ca and P in the peritubular as in the intertubular matrix, although they could not determine a statistical difference in the P $K\alpha \cdot$ Ca $K\alpha^3$ ratio found in these two areas.

Johnson and Singer (*95*) investigated with the electron microprobe the distribution of strontium in incisors from rats fed low (0.0002%) or high (0.45%) Sr for 43 days. Data obtained indicated that strontium produced a decreased mineralization and an inverse relationship between strontium and calcium content. In incisors from rats fed the high level of strontium, a gradient of increasing strontium concentrations from the incisal to apical areas was observed. The phosphorus content was relatively constant throughout the enamel.

The chemical changes produced in the tooth as the advancing front of caries demineralization progresses into the dentin have been studied by Suga *et al.* (*187*). They reported that magnesium was one of the first elements to be lowered in concentration. Frank, Capitant, and Goni (*58*) used a new approach to make the density of the sample uniform by substituting the organic matter with the soluble salt KI. They compared the superficial enamel layer of caries-resistant and caries-susceptible enamel and found no significant differences in the distribution of calcium and phosphorus in the two groups. Chloride is more concentrated in the superficial enamel layer, decreases toward the dentinoenamel junction, and does not show any statistical difference in concentration between these two groups of teeth. Initial carious lesions were studied with the electron probe, and the loss of Ca and P in the subsurface was confirmed, especially along the striae of Retzius, but the superficial caries layer had a normal Cl, Ca, and P content.

Frazier (*59*) used the electron probe also to study the distribution of Ca and P in incipient carious lesions in human teeth. His findings indicated that the superficial layer was either hypermineralized or hypomineralized when compared with normal enamel of the same tooth. The Ca/P ratios in the outer layer of the lesion did not vary significantly from values obtained from normal unaltered enamel. One of the most interesting observations was that the Ca/P molar ratio indicated that the lowest ratios were associated with the highest phosphorus intensities in the hypermineralized areas. The lowest phosphorus intensities and highest ratios were associated with hypomineralized areas; thus, although low in both calcium and phosphorus, the hypomineralized areas were disproportionately low in phosphorus.

Teeth which had been treated with stannous fluoride were analyzed with the electron probe by Hoerman *et al.* (*86*). They reported that tin was randomly distributed on the enamel surface in selected areas of enrichment of about 125 $\mu$ in diameter and 20 $\mu$ deep. This suggests that tin uptake may take place in selected areas such as the "white spots." Further work in this area using the electron probe should yield information of great value to understanding the progression of enamel caries, the uptake of topical cariostatic compounds, and, probably what is most important, the process of post-eruptive maturation of enamel.

Brudevold *et al.* (*30*) studied the composition and distribution of minerals in dental tissues in relation to enamel maturation. Enamel maturation has been discussed often in the literature, but little is known in detail about the processes involved. The studies of these investigators on mineral composition and distribution in enamel indicates "that changes occurring in the enamel after it is calcified are confined to the outer portion and that these changes to a great extent are concerned with surface accumulation of trace elements. It is suggested that maturation involves these surface changes."

**Pre-Eruptive and Post-Eruptive Mineralization (Maturation).** Deakins (*50*) in 1942 in a classical study investigated the pre-eruptive changes in the enamel which increase its hardness from the initial time of deposition to the eruption of the tooth. These changes are mainly in terms of an increased mineralization and density and a concomitant loss of water from the tooth mineral portion.

When the tooth erupts into the oral cavity it is highly mineralized, but at the same time certain surfaces are highly reactive. Recently erupted teeth, when exposed to such bone-seekers as murexide, will be intensively stained, while teeth that have been exposed to the oral environment for a longer period will not take up the stain. The changes that take place in the enamel surface after the tooth has erupted constitute the post-eruptive maturation process. The reactivity of the mineral decreases with age and varies with its immediate environment, structure, and chemical composition. Scott *et al.* (*165*) reported that there is a progressive decrease in visible structures on the surfaces of teeth from individuals of increasing ages. This loss of structural detail may possibly reflect a deposit of mineral substances in rough areas and scratches.

Saliva mediates this mineralizing effect on erupted teeth. More than 50 years ago, Head (*76*) observed that when teeth are softened by demineralization they can be rehardened by immersion in fresh saliva. The remineralization phenomenon is, therefore, to some extent the converse of dental caries and represents a natural phenomenon in the oral cavity. Brudevold and Messer (*25*) demonstrated that salivary sediment and apatite crystals can act as matrices to initiate calcification and catalyze crystal formation. The mineral formation induced by hydroxyapatite was greatly accelerated in the presence of fluoride ions (0.2 ppm). Similar results have been reported by Pigman (*149*), who studied the conditions controlling the rehardening of human enamel *in vitro*. Fluoride was present in all cases and seemed to play an important role in the calcification process.

Using polarizing microscopy and microradiography, Johansson (*93*) observed that the remineralization of acid-etched ground sections of enamel is rapid during the first 24 hours and does not change much, even after several weeks' exposure to the calcifying solutions of parotid saliva. Examination with the polarizing microscope revealed a decrease in opacity due to the deposition of mineral in the outer enamel. The remineralized surface was relatively impermeable, since very light staining was observed when it was immersed in a saturated solution of alizarin C red stain, while the control etched enamel was markedly stained.

Ericsson (*55*) has shown that carious lesions in teeth avidly take up radioactive Ca and P. Von der Fehr (*202*) also has shown *in vitro* and *in vivo* the uptake of minerals from saliva into the enamel lesions. These investigations strongly suggest that there is a dynamic balance at the tooth surface in which trace elements may play a fundamental role. When demineralizing agents become extremely active and remineralization is unable to repair the damaged site, a mineral imbalance takes place which may tip the equilibrium toward dental caries. In the rat, molars show areas of hypomineralized enamel at the time of eruption (*57, 187*) which disappear with time if the animals are maintained on a noncariogenic diet (*22, 23, 177*). The regression of these hypomineralized areas which constitute the post-eruptive maturation is important in the prevention of caries and is influenced to a great extent by the mineral environment around the teeth.

A final thought with regard to these two very distinct periods in the life of the tooth should be stressed. Incorporation of a trace element can take place pre-eruptively in a diffuse way throughout the tooth structure with higher concentrations in the dentin near the pulp and external enamel; it can concentrate primarily on the surface of enamel just after eruption, and also during the maturation period until that time when the tooth mineral becomes practically unavailable for reaction; and it can accumulate at certain sites of chemical erosion or etched enamel surfaces which then become highly reactive.

### *Influence of Minerals on Dental Caries*

Information with regard to the chemical composition of teeth, the effects of food ashes on dental caries, and the epidemiological investigations has stimulated interest in the effects of individual trace elements on dental caries (*1, 34, 72, 106*). Reports on this subject present conflicting results which confuse their interpretation. The information we have at present allows only a tentative classification of the elements according to their capability to promote or reduce caries in experimental animals into five groups:

(1) Caries-promoting elements: Se, Mg, Cd, Pt, Pb, Si.
(2) Elements that are mildly cariostatic: Mo, V, Sr, Cu, B, Li, Au.
(3) Elements with doubtful effect on caries: Be, Co, Mn, Sn, Zn, Br, I.

(4) Caries-inert elements: Ba, Al, Ni, Fe, Pd, Ti.

(5) Elements that are strongly cariostatic: F, P.

This last group has been discussed previously in this monograph, so the evaluation will be done only on the first four groups.

**Caries-Promoting Elements.** SELENIUM. Selenium is closely related chemically to sulfur and tellurium. Moxon (*119*) conducted extensive studies of the toxic effects of Se in animals (alkali disease). It was not until Schwarz (*162*) identified *Factor 3* as a Se-containing compound which gave complete protection against dietary liver necrosis in the rat that Se was considered an essential element in human nutrition (*163, 164*).

The first observation with regard to the effect of Se on dentition came from Smith and Westfall (*170*), who reported a high incidence of "poor teeth" in seleniferous areas. Wheatcroft *et al.* (*206*) administered Na selenite intraperitoneally to adult rats and observed no significant effect on dentition; however, a marked toxic action was noted when 0.5 and 1.0 mg of Se per kg body weight were given. At the higher level, there was a trend (insignificant at the 1% level) toward increased caries incidence.

Hadjimarkos (*68, 71*) carried out epidemiological studies in Oregon among children 14–16 years of age residing in 10 counties. The prevalence of dental caries and mean levels of urinary Se concentration among children living in four of these counties is tabulated in Table V.

**Table V. Dental Caries *vs.* Urinary Se**

| *County (Oregon)* | *DMF Teeth/Child* | *Urinary Se Concentration, Ppm* |
|---|---|---|
| Klamath | 9.0 | 0.037 |
| Clatsop | 14.4 | 0.049 |
| Jackson | 13.4 | 0.074 |
| Josephine | 14.4 | 0.076 |

Hadjimarkos reported a positive correlation between the concentration of urinary Se and dental caries prevalence.

Tank and Storvick (*190*) carried out a similar investigation in areas known to be seleniferous and in control areas where no seleniferous soils existed. Dental examinations were made of children 10–18 years of age who had been born and lived in the two areas, demonstrating a higher incidence of caries in those from seleniferous areas. Unfortunately, there was an inadequate sampling procedure in collecting urine specimens and the Se levels of urinary excretion could not be determined. Cadell and Cousins (*37*), working in New Zealand, found no significant difference between urinary Se levels of school boys 5 to 14 years of age and their caries prevalence. The Se concentrations found among the New Zealand children were below those found in the Oregon county children who showed the lowest level of urinary Se concentration.

The experimental animal studies in relation to selenium have shown contradictory results. English (*54*) described hypoplastic changes in the enamel of female dogs treated with thiouracil or organic Se. Muhler and Shafer (*127*) pointed out that Se suppresses thyroid activity and may be compared with thiouracil, which increases caries. The activity of the thyroid gland appears to be related to the incidence of dental caries in the rat, for injected thyroxine significantly decreases dental caries, whereas radiothyroidectomy significantly increases it (*123*). Muhler and Shafer (*126*) fed Na selenite (15–30 ppm in a corn caries-promoting diet) to young rats and noted no effect on dental caries development or in the histology of the salivary glands. The growth of rats was about half that of the controls, and, therefore, the toxic effect may have obscured the dental effect of selenium.

Buttner (*36*) offered rats diets containing lower levels of Na selenite (5–10 ppm) in the drinking water and obtained a 38 and 54% increase in carious lesions as well as decreased reproduction and decreased weight gain. These toxic effects were reported also by Muhlemann and Konig (*120*) when distilled water containing 3.3 ppm of selenium as $SeO_2$ was offered to weanling rats during a short 20-day experimental period. The impaired growth of rats on selenium was accompanied by a caries inhibition. In this same experiment, they tested V (2.1 ppm), Pt (8.0 ppm), Au (6.8 ppm), and $SnCl_3$ (0.1%) and found them all without effect.

Because the effectiveness of fluorides in reducing dental caries has been related to the degree to which they are concentrated in the enamel, some investigators have evaluated selenium incorporation into oral tissues. Claycomb *et al.* (*40*) investigated the uptake of $Se^{75}$ by salivary glands, teeth, and saliva of the rat following intracardiac administration. While the salivary glands are permeable to Se, they do not accumulate this element. Selenium activity in teeth seemed to parallel that of the salivary glands. Thomassen and Leicester (*193*) injected intraperitoneally radioactive $Se^{75}$ in rats and followed the incorporation of selenium into several tissues in a longitudinal study. Selenium appeared to have been deposited in all tissues, with the lung and the kidney containing the largest amount in rats sacrificed four days after the injection. The Se levels in molars and incisors were lower than in any other tissues and dropped even lower after the first four days but maintained this low level in molars for a very long period of time (182 days). Hadjimarkos and Bonhorst (*70*) reported that Se is present in low concentrations in enamel and dentin from human teeth. Autoradiographic studies done in our laboratories indicate that $Se^{75}$ fed in the diet of rats as sodium selenite was found abundantly in the pulp and extravascular areas of teeth, but also in lower concentrations in the mineralized portions of the teeth, which probably accounts for the selenium found by Thomassen and Leicester after a long experimental period.

If selenium does not accumulate to a large extent in the superficial layers of enamel, such as is the case with fluoride, then other mechanisms must be investigated. Claycomb *et al.* (*41*) investigated the effect of dietary sodium selenite (4.56 ppm Se) on dental caries of rats and found no significant difference in caries incidence between test and control, in an experiment lasting 100 days. Navia *et al.* (*135*) investigated the caries activity of 4 ppm Se as $Na_2SeO_3$ in the drinking water or in the purified caries promoting diet #200 (Navia *et al.*, *134*) and found that Se was without effect, except upon sulcal lesions in groups fed Se in the drinking water. Hadjimarkos (*67*) advanced the suggestion that disturbances in the regulation of food or water intake resulting from the addition of the Se supplement may be the factor which influences the degree of cariogenicity of the diet. Our results indicate that even though there is a decrease in food intake of the group offered the Se in the water, the cariogenic action is only significant in the sulcal caries and not in the smooth buccal or the proximal surfaces. These results point more to an effect of the selenium on the oral flora, and preliminary observations indicate to us that this is a possibility.

In conclusion, there is evidence from both epidemiological and animal studies that selenium has a slight caries-promoting property, but further work should be done to elucidate the mechanism of action of Se on dental caries and to differentiate its toxic effects from those which are physiological.

MAGNESIUM. The adult human body contains approximately 25 grams of magnesium (*207*), of which 70% is associated with calcium and phosphorus in bone and teeth salts. Magnesium is present in both enamel and dentin, but its concentration in the latter is usually twice that in enamel. Magnesium, a divalent cation like calcium, does not replace it in the apatite crystal; rather, it is considered to be confined to the surface positions (*136*). The effect of magnesium on the precipitation of calcium carbonates and phosphates *in vitro* has been investigated by Bachra *et al.* (*9*). Their results indicated that magnesium stabilized the amorphous precipitates of calcium carbonates and phosphates and also disturbed the crystallization of the apatite. Apatitic precipitates were more poorly crystallized when formed in the presence of Mg ions than when formed in their absence.

Magnesium is one of the principal cations of soft tissues where it is found as an intracellular element. The essentiality of magnesium in plant nutrition has been known for many years and its presence in the porphyrin moeity of chlorophyll has stimulated numerous investigations concerning its function in green plants. In animal tissues, its first-discovered and probable major role is that of enzyme activator such as in the case of the phosphatases and the enzymes of the glycolytic systems. Both of these enzyme systems have a major role in the calcification and decalcification processes of teeth.

Irving (*88*) investigated the influence of diets low in magnesium upon the histological appearance of the incisor tooth of the rat and described the alterations of the calcification rhythm as well as the adventitious calcification occurring in the deficient state. Beck and Furuta (*13*) studied the effect of Mg-deficient diets on oral and dental tissues and concluded that this element is an essential mineral for enamel formation in the rat. Yamame (*216*), working with hamsters to which a diet containing a low level of Mg (40 ppm) was offered, observed a marked resorption of alveolar bone, widening of the periodontal ligament space, as well as disorganization of collagen fibers. These findings suggest that magnesium has an important role in the development and maintenance of the tooth and its supporting structures.

In 1948, McClure published a summary of results of various modifications of food and drinking water offered to rats. Addition of 500 ppm of Mg as $MgCl_2$ to the water increased caries. McClure and McCann (*115*) drastically altered the Ca, P, and Mg levels of a diet offered to weanling white rats for periods of approximately 60 days. Rather than reducing caries, the $MgCO_3$ supplement increased the caries severity score. Hendershot and Forsaith (*82*) observed that caries scores were increased three-fold when rats were fed a magnesium salt of ethylenediaminetetraacetic acid (Mg-EDTA). Forbes (*56*) noted that Mg salts did not affect the production of acid in saliva. Toth (*196*) observed that the mean magnesium content of saliva was three times higher in caries-resistant than in caries-active gypsies (1.59 mg *vs.* 0.52 mg Mg/100 ml).

Richie (*153*) reported that he was able to increase the magnesium content of human teeth by feeding a mixture of magnesium and calcium phosphates and a small percentage of potassium, sodium, and iron phosphates. He associated this increase in magnesium with caries resistance but used too few subjects to permit statistical analysis and confused his results by using phosphates which have cariostatic properties.

Navia *et al.* (*132*) studied the effect of dietary magnesium supplements fed to rats at a level of 2000 ppm in a factorial study. Sulcal and smooth carious lesions were high in groups receiving the Mg supplement, low in those given the trimetaphosphate, and decreased further when magnesium and the condensed phosphate were fed together, demonstrating a strong significant interaction. These results were further confirmed in a larger factorial study (Navia *et al.*, *131*) involving two elements besides these, zinc and manganese, which have no effect on dental caries scores of rats offered these supplements in the diet at a 2000 ppm level.

Parma *et al.* (*147*) reported that the cariostatic effect of F is enhanced when Mg is added to the drinking water. The relationship of magnesium to tooth growth, development, and maintenance, as well as its influence on the cariostatic effects of compounds such as fluorides and phosphate, is the object of research in our laboratories. The understanding of these relationships should be important to oral health programs in the future, for magnesium may have a beneficial or detrimental effect, depending on the level in the diet and the time of feeding.

CADMIUM. Little is really known about the possible role of Cd in the metabolism of bones and teeth. Ginn and Volker (*61*) reported that 50 ppm $CdCl_3$ added to a rice diet reduced the pigmentation of the enamel of rat incisors and caused anemia, but did not reduce dental caries. When the same level was added to the drinking water, caries were stimulated. Pindborg *et al.* (*150*) confirmed the observation on incisor enamel pigmentation. An increase in caries was noted (*102*) when 20 and 40 ppm of $CdCl_3$ were added to the drinking water of rats. Wisotzky and Hein (*210, 211*) repeated the observation of incisor depigmentation and also noted a bleaching of the fur and severe anemia in hamsters fed 0.5 meq $CdSO_4$. This level of $CdSO_4$ increased the caries by 11% in male, and 99% in female hamsters (*212*). Parizek (*145, 146*) noted that subcutaneously-injected Cd salts destroyed testicular tissues, but not when large excesses of zinc acetate were given simultaneously. This may indicate that an interrelationship exists between these two elements for some active site in an enzyme system. Bird and Thomas (15) observed that Cd inhibited *in vitro* mineralization and apatite crystal formation, and this may relate to its cariogenic properties.

PLATINUM. Platinum, as platinic chloride, accelerated caries to the point that the dentition was destroyed almost completely (*209, 210*). Hein *et al.* (*77, 79*) found platinic chloride to be cariogenic.

LEAD. Lead, as lead acetate, caused an acceleration of caries in hamsters (*210*).

**Elements That Are Mildly Cariostatic.** MOLYBDENUM. Molybdenum is required for the maintenance of normal levels of xanthine oxidase in the liver and intestine of the rat. It is also a part of liver aldehyde oxidase (another flavoprotein) which catalyzes the oxidation of aldehydes. It is an essential mineral element for higher animals. Adler and Straub (*3*) reported that the incidence of caries in populations living in certain Hungarian towns was lower than would be expected from the F content of the water supply, and deduced that it was because of its Mo content (0.1 ppm). Adler (*2*) noted a definite beneficial effect on caries when rats were fed 0.10 ppm Mo. Hadjimarkos (*66*) stated that the total amount of Mo ingested should be considered rather than the amount found in the water, and this is a valid point. Ludwig (*107*) found that 6-, 7-, and 8-year-old children in Napier (New Zealand) had 57, 46, and 21%, respectively, fewer carious teeth than similar children in Hastings. Later, it was reported (*108*) that this effect was related to the Mo content of the foods grown in the area, possibly in association with other elements. Jenkins (*90, 91, 92*) reviewed the epidemiological studies as well as the investigations dealing with molybdenum interactions with other elements and the *in vitro* experiments and concluded that this element has mild cariostatic properties which deserve the attention of dental investigators.

The interrelations between Mo and other elements have been studied by several investigators. Crane (*45*) observed that Mo increased the intestinal absorption of F. Stookey and Muhler (*181*) found that Mo increased the retention of F by the rat. Less F was excreted by the group receiving the Mo supplement. Buttner (*35, 36*), however, did not observe increased F retention by the femurs when rats were fed F and Mo together. When 50 ppm Mo were given in the drinking water, there was no increase in bone fluoride. He concluded that the cariostatic action observed when Mo and F were given together cannot be explained in terms of increased F utilization by concomitant ingestion of Mo. Van Reen, Ostrom, and Berzinskas (*199*) also observed no effect when 10 ppm of Mo were fed in the diet as Na molybdate to NMRI-D rats during gestation and lactation and subsequently for 5 weeks to the weanling rats, when weanling rats were fed a purified, caries-promoting diet with supplements up to 48 ppm Mo, or when weanling rats were given up to 24 ppm F in the drinking water together with 24 ppm Mo, in which case only the F contribution was noted. These investigators (*200*) reported further experiments confirming their previous findings and pointed out that the negligible protective effect of molybdenum in the NMRI-D rat may be related to this strain's high caries activity, which is usually several times larger than in animals used in other studies (*108, 182*).

Malthus *et al.* (*111*) reported that there is a strong synergistic effect when Mo and F are supplemented together in the drinking water of rats at a 25 ppm level, but no significant effect when Mo is fed alone at the 25 ppm level. During the conduct of this experiment, changes had to be made in the levels of Cu, Zn, and Mn in the purified cariogenic diet which may have obscured the final results.

Bowen and Eastoe (*18*) studied the effect of sugar solutions containing 10–60 ppm fluoride and 10–60 ppm molybdenum on the pH of plaque in monkeys and reported that Mo, when used at the same concentration, was not as effective as fluoride in preventing acid production. Jenkins' work (*92*) is in agreement with this, although they differ in that he found the greatest effect on human saliva at pH 5.0 while in monkeys the greatest effect was observed in the higher pH range. Jenkins' work suggests that the effectiveness of Mo may reside in its capacity to reduce salivary acid production. Other investigators (*99*) studied the possible effect of molybdenum (and fluoride, also) on tooth morphology but failed to see significant alterations except for the fact that fluoride and the interaction of F and Mo altered significantly the widths of the fissures and the thickness of enamel and dentin lining the fissures. Kruger (*100*) had previously conducted a statistically designed experiment, and observed that Mo injected into rats daily from the 5th to the 17th day after birth at a level of 2 to 7 μg a day produced a significant reduction in dental caries, so tooth morphology does not seem to be a factor in the cariostatic mechanism. Shaw and Griffiths (*168*) noted some reduction in rat caries when ammonium molybdate was fed post-developmentally (100–200 ppm), but no effect when fed during the development of the molars. Ammonium paramolybdate, however, had no effect post-developmentally and increased caries when fed during development.

Mo appears promising as a cariostatic agent, and the indication exists that its caries-reducing properties are exhibited at levels below its toxic dose. No attention has been paid to the interaction that other elements such as Cu, W, and the sulfate ion have with Mo. These would influence profoundly the biological activity of molybdenum. The evidence is still inadequate, and further work should be carried out.

VANADIUM. Trace amounts of V are distributed widely in both soils and vegetation. This element resembles P in chemical behavior.

Rygh (*160, 161*) prepared a highly purified diet, added different mineral elements to it, and observed that Sr, Ba, Zn, Tl, and V are nutrient essentials for rats and guinea pigs. He concluded that of these V and Sr promoted calcification during the growth of bones and teeth, while excess Ba, Zn, and Tl all cause decreased calcification. When Sr and V were absent, caries increased; when present, caries was controlled. Deletion of Zn, Ba, and Tl from the diet had no effect on dental caries.

This result prompted Geyer (*60*) to test V in small groups of hamsters. Markedly less enamel caries was observed in hamsters fed daily 0.08 mg $V_2O_5$ in comparison with controls on the cariogenic diet, and dentinal caries also was stopped. He suggested that ". . . vanadium ions, imbedded in enamel and dentin, could increase the hardness of the hydroxyl apatite as well as the cohesion between the organic and inorganic matter."

Hein and Witsotzky (*81*) found no inhibition of caries in hamsters that had been given 10 ppm V in the drinking water. An increase in caries was noted when slightly higher amounts were given. This is a toxic level of intake. Muhler (*121*) fed 10, 20, and 40 μg of vanadium pentoxide per cc in the drinking water of rats and noted no effect on caries when these high toxic levels of V were given.

The concentration of V given seems to be important. Winiker (*208*) fed a salt of ammonium metavanadate to hamsters and noted caries inhibition when 0.035 mg/day were fed and caries stimulation when 0.20 mg/day were given.

Munch (*128*) observed favorable results when both V and Mo were given. He postulated that V acts locally on the teeth by changing the lattice of the hydroxyl apatite, with V replacing P.

Kruger (*100*) confirmed Geyer in a study on rats begun during amelogenesis in the rat. Rat molar caries were reduced significantly. However, Shaw and Griffiths (*168*) observed no effect when vanadium pentoxide or vanadyl sulfate was fed in the diet or in the drinking water. There was uncertainty in the results when the V salts were fed during the developmental stage.

The studies by Tank and Storvick (*190*) on children from seleniferous and nonseleniferous areas indicate an inverse correlation between the V content of the water and caries development.

Some studies have been made of the interrelationship between F and V. Tempestini (*191*) noted that F and V together were more effective in reducing dental caries than F alone. Buttner (*36*) did not confirm this finding.

V deserves further investigation to determine its effects on bone and tooth calcification and on dental caries development.

STRONTIUM. This bone-seeking alkaline earth metal appears to affect caries. Shaw and Griffiths (*168*) noted no evidence of vanadium reducing dental caries incidence. Rygh (*158, 159*) noted a high incidence of caries when Sr was absent from the diet of rats. When Sr and V were added in plenty, caries was curtailed. Johansen and Hein (*94*) concluded that 50 ppm of strontium as $SrCl_2$ added to drinking water had no effect on hamsters' caries.

Banks *et al.* (*10*) reported that 1.0 to 2.0% $SrCl_2$ added to the drinking water of weanling rats caused considerable disturbances of the calcification of the dentin and cementum. Pindborg (*151*) made a similar observation, and noted a lack of pigmentation of the normal enamel of the rat incisor. Steadman *et al.* (*178*) suggested that Sr is deposited primarily before the eruption and during the calcification of the tooth, though additional Sr is deposited in the secondary dentin and cementum after tooth eruption. Therefore, children will deposit considerable amounts of $Sr^{90}$ when there is heavy isotope fallout. Bryant *et al.* (*32*) corroborated this conclusion, for they found an inverse correlation with age. Butler (*33*) found $2.6 \pm 0.6$ disintegrations of $Sr^{90}$/min/gram in teeth obtained from children under 4 years and $0.4 \pm 0.2$ in teeth from human subjects over 31 years of age.

Yaeger (*215*) observed by the use of an electron microscope that the matrix of the fine structure of the hypomineralized component produced by Sr contained pools of heavily stained homogeneous, interfibrillar material, presumably nonfibrillar collagen. This defect probably could account for the inhibition of mineralization which results in the hypomineralized component of the incisors studied.

Further studies of the role of Sr in calcification and in dental caries are needed.

COPPER. Copper, an essential element, is a constituent or an activator of certain enzymes, and it has a postulated role in bone formation and in maintenance of myelin within the nervous system. Crippling bone defects occur in cattle and sheep grazing on Cu-deficient pastures.

Brudevold and Steadman (*26*) studied the distribution of Cu in human teeth, and found no correlation between Cu content and tooth pigmentation or caries. McClure (*113*) found no pronounced caries effect when Cu was given in drinking water. Shaw (*167*) noted no effect when 0.5% Na–Cu chlorophyllin was added to the drinking water of rats. However, Hein and Shafer (*80*), using a preparation of Na–Cu chlorophyllin of 93.2% purity, found a cariostatic effect in hamsters.

Concentrations of 0.25 mg/100 grams Cu in sucrose-containing saliva definitely inhibited acid formation while 3 to 4 mg/100 grams Cu in saliva completely inhibited acid production (*56*). Dreizen *et al.* (*52*) found no relation between the Cu content of saliva and dental caries activity in human subjects. The level of Cu normally present in saliva was unable *in vitro* to prevent the growth of *L. acidophilus*.

Hein (*78*) observed that $CuSO_4$ reduced caries as the level was increased: 0, 10, 25, 50 ppm Cu. A straight line was obtained when the caries scores were plotted against the logarithm of the Cu concentration, indicating that tooth destruction was an inverse function of the $CuSO_4$ concentration. Kruger (*100*) injected 0.005 to 0.02 mg of $CuNO_3$ intraperitoneally into rats, and noted a caries reduction which approached the 5% significance level.

BORON. This was the first element to be proved essential for plant life. It is not clear yet whether it is an essential element for animals.

Wessinger (*205*) gave 200 mg B/kg body weight as boric acid and observed no enamel hypoplasia in the incisors. He concluded that B had no effect on amelogenesis in contrast to Sr which has a marked effect. Kruger (*100*) gave 0.005 to 0.025 mg B as boric acid intraperitoneally, and concluded that B is effective in reducing caries development. Shaw *et al.* (*168*) noted a modest reduction in caries when 0.5, 1.0, and 2.0% Na borate were fed post-developmentally.

LITHIUM. Wisotzky and Hein (*210*) tested lithium sulfate and found no effect on animal caries. However, Shaw and Griffiths (*168*) added a 0.1% supplement of lithium carbonate to a rats' diet and observed a definite post-developmental influence to inhibit dental caries.

GOLD. Gold, in the form of auric chloride, was reported by Wisotzky and Hein (*210*) to be a potent inhibitor of caries in hamsters.

**Elements With Doubtful Caries Effect.** BERYLLIUM. This alkaline earth metal has been reported to produce changes in both bones and teeth. Maynard *et al.* (*112*) fed weanling rats a diet containing 5% $BeSO_4$ or $BeCO_3$ and observed rachitic lesions within 3 weeks. Wentz (*204*) fed 3 and 6% levels of $BeCO_3$ and observed rickets if the vitamin D intake was low, as well as enamel hypoplasia and aplasia, retardation in calcification and in dentin formation, and delayed eruption of the teeth. Sherman and Sobel (*169*) reported that extremely low concentrations (0.01 ppm) of Be ion can limit calcium phosphate crystal growth, and this might explain the *in vivo* results. Rygh (*161*) concluded that while F is essential to the proper formation of tooth enamel, Be is of no significance.

Leicester *et al.* (*103*) found that when male hamsters were given 0.02% $BeCl_2$ in diet or in drinking water from the date of conception until 24 days postpartum, a highly significant reduction in dental decay was observed 100 days later. These authors noted (*192*) that when Fe and F were fed together to male hamsters, there was a statistically significant reduction in caries.

COBALT. Cobalt is a constituent of vitamin $B_{12}$ which affects blood formation, but no definite relation between $B_{12}$ deficiency and caries has been observed. Dreizen *et al.* (*52*) found no relation between the Co level in saliva of human beings and their caries experience. Hendershot and Forsaith (*82*) found 3 to 4 times more caries in male rats fed a supplement of Co-EDTA salt than in controls.

Cobalt may interfere with the mineralization process, for Goldenberg (*63*) noted that the addition of Co (also Be, Mn, Ni) to a basal solution which contained NaCl, KCl, and $NaHCO_3$ accelerated the inactivation of the calcifying mechanism of an epiphyseal cartilage suspended in the solution. Bird and Thomas (*15*) found Co unique in preventing the formation of apatite crystals at concentrations which also inhibited mineralization of rachitic cartilage matrix.

MANGANESE. Manganese is an activator for several enzymes such as blood and bone phosphatases. It is an essential element even though there is no definite evidence that Mn deficiency occurs in man.

Stephan and Harris (*180*) noted that dental caries was somewhat high when Mn was omitted from a synthetic-type diet, and reduced when 0.1% Mn was added. Wynn *et al.* (*215*) added 50, 150, and 500 ppm of Mn to the synthetic type diets of rats and noted no caries-reducing effect. Similar experiments by Hendershot and Forsaith (*82*) with the

Mn salt of ethylenediaminetetraacetic acid, Mn acetate, or Mn versenate were also negative. When 0.15 mg Mn, as the sulfate, was injected intraperitoneally daily into rats, the caries incidence did not decrease (*100*). Navia *et al.* (*131*) studied the effect of $MnCl_2$ supplements (2000 ppm $Mn^{2+}$) on a purified caries-promoting diet fed to rats and found no effect on caries.

Dreizen *et al.* (*51*) showed that the conversion of carbohydrates to acid residues by oral bacteria is inhibited when $Mn^{2+}$ is removed by chelating compounds. They suggested that the Mn content of the saliva, which approximates 0.005 $\mu$g/ml, could be an important factor in dental caries activity. Buttner (*36*) found no interaction between Mn and F metabolism, even though El Tannir (*53*) had suggested that the results of an epidemiological survey in Mecca indicated that Mn caused a brown coloration of the mottled enamel in human subjects consuming water containing 2 ppm F.

It is evident that the caries activity of Mn is still unclear.

TIN. Tin has been studied extensively in recent years, especially in relation to F. Muhler and Day (*124*) supplemented the drinking water of rats with 10 ppm SnF and found it superior to NaF in reducing the incidence and severity of dental caries, while $SnCl_2$ had no significant effect. They observed (*125*) a 75% decrease in caries incidence when it was fed in the diet of rats. Toxic effects were noted when 500 ppm were fed, as shown by growth impairment. Sn gluconate and $SnCl_2$ were essentially without effect (*121*), but $SnF_2$ had a greater effect than corresponded to its fluoride content. Muhler (*122*) suggested that the most significant clinical effect of topically-applied $SnF_2$ is exerted on incipient lesions, and Meckel (*117*) indicated that tin is held very firmly and no significant losses take place for periods up to 113 days. The work of Hoerman *et al.* (*86*) with the electron probe microanalysis indicates that the mechanism of this long persistence of tin might be its special binding properties in "enriched" areas of enamel, from which it is leached slowly over a long period of time.

Gish *et al.* (*62*) treated 442 children with a 4% aqueous solution of K fluorostannite and found a 53.7% reduction in DMFT and a 39.2% reduction in DMFS. Brudevold *et al.* (*29*) reported that $Sn^{2+}$ and $F^-$ were both taken up when the enamel was exposed to $SnF_2$ solutions, especially when the pH was low.

ZINC. Zinc is present in bone (*194*) and is quite high in dentin (*46*, *47*). Increased levels have been reported in the dental tissues of tuberculosis patients. It is distributed widely in the human body, especially in the erythrocytes where it is an essential component of carbonic anhydrase. Zinc is also a structural component of the phosphatases, to which it contributes stability. Zinc accumulates on the surface structures of the teeth (*31*), but occurs in low concentrations in subsurface material, and shows a distribution pattern similar to F and Pb. It is a dietary essential (*161*).

Little is known about the effects of Zn on dental caries. McClure (*113*) noted a caries-stimulating effect when $ZnSO_4$ (250 ppm) was fed in the drinking water of rats. Hendershot and Forsaith (*82, 83*) observed appreciably lower caries scores when Zn-EDTA was fed to weanling male rats, but no significant effect when Zn acetate was given. Zn supplements as $ZnCl_2$ (2000 ppm $Zn^{2+}$) offered to rats from birth to 60 days of age were inert in terms of smooth surface and sulcal caries (*131*).

BROMINE. Bromine, when fed as the bromide, was found by Sognnaes (*171*) to increase caries in rats when fed during tooth development, but to reduce caries somewhat if fed after eruption. Using serial autoradiography and $Br^{82}$, Soremark (*174*) showed that bromide ions enter the dentin and that its action may vary, depending on the period when administered.

IODINE. Iodine (0.005 to 0.002 mg) injected intraperitoneally into rats had no effect on caries (*100*). Several investigators (*49, 114, 152*) have found that compounds like iodoacetic acid cause a significant reduction in caries when added to drinking water. Dale and Keyes (*48*) observed an additive effect when iodoacetic acid was given with fluorine. Unfortunately, the $LD_{50}$ of iodoacetic acid is 116 ± 12 mg/kg body weight, which gives a safety margin that is too narrow to permit its application as propyhlactic agent for caries (*110*).

SILICON. Silicon oils are cariogenic when fed in the diet at 10 and 20% levels (*20*), but silicofluoride salts have been used successfully for fluoridation of water supplies without any apparent reduction in the effectiveness of the fluoride in reducing caries. No evidence has been presented indicating that Si is caries-promoting in humans.

**Caries-Inert Elements.** BARIUM. When 0.5 or 1.0% of $BaCl_2$ was fed in the diet of rats, it had no effect on the developing teeth or caries susceptibility (*168*); however, some reduction in caries was observed post-developmentally. No alteration in the rate or degree of calcification in these animals was observed.

ALUMINUM. This element is abundant in the soil, and is ubiquitous in foods, but is not known to be essential to higher animals. Its toxicity is quite low.

Wynn and Haldi (*213*) noted no effect on experimental caries development in rats when 0.16, 2.0, and 20 ppm Al were added to the diet. Kruger (*100*) found no effect on rat caries when 0.008 and 0.025 mg of Al were fed as Al acetate. Similar negative results were reported by Van Reen *et al.* (*200*).

It appears to counteract dental fluorosis (*201, 203*). This effect is probably a result of decreased deposition of F, since the F stores in bones and teeth were reduced by concurrent Al feeding.

NICKEL. Nickel is widely distributed in plant and animal tissues. It acts as an activator of several enzyme systems, such as arginase and trypsin.

Forbes and Smith (*56*) found that Ni salts exert a marked inhibiting action on acid production in saliva. Hendershot *et al.* (*83*) reported that $NiCl_2$ caused an increase of caries in rats, that when Ni-EDTA was given, caries was inhibited in male but not in female rats, and that Ni acetate had no effect on either sex.

IRON. This element is important to hemoglobin formation and is an essential element. Though normally it is not considered a part of the apatite molecule, it appears essential for the formation of the orange-brown pigment that is characteristic of the enamel of the rodent incisors.

McClure (*113*) fed 250 and 500 ppm ferric citrate in the diet of rats and noted no distinct effect. The same result was reported by Wynn *et al.* (*215*) and by Hendershot and Forsaith (*82*) when fed Fe-EDTA. Torell (*195*) suggested the possibility that ferric solutions may establish layers of hydrolized ferric precipitates on enamel which could increase caries.

PALADIUM. Paladium chloride had no effect on caries (*210*).

TITANIUM. Van Reen *et al.* (*200*) found this element to be caries-inert when tested with the NMRI-D rats, although a small reduction (about 10%) was observed when Al, Ti, and Mo were fed together in the diet.

### *Experimental Factors Which Contribute to the Discrepancy in the Effect of Minerals on Dental Caries*

The reviewed results of a large number of experiments in humans and animals to investigate the relationship between certain trace elements and dental caries are conflicting. The reason for this apparent confusion is primarily that many factors are involved in this problem. Experiments in which only some of the factors are taken into consideration cannot be compared with other experiments where a different set of factors has been controlled.

In order to clarify this point, it would be of advantage to review briefly the experimental factors which influence dental caries research with regard to trace elements.

**Species.** The sensitivity of animal species to the effect of certain elements has a wide variation, owing principally to their anatomical, biochemical, physiological, and microbiological differences. These differences are not only present within animal species (rats, hamsters, monkeys) and even strains, but also between animal species and human beings, making the extrapolation of results a difficult task. The animal is an experimental model, where assumptions have to be made and, therefore, results from this type of study can only be used to understand better the pathology of human caries, and not to explain in its entirety the human caries phenomena.

**Route of Administration.** Elements can influence the tooth and its environment by entering the organism through diet, water, air, or cage environment. Experimentally, elements also can be administered by injection and by topical applications on the tooth surface (*73*). The effectiveness of these different routes in facilitating the effect of the chemical agent is dependent on the availability of the compound and its particular mechanism of action on the tooth—*i.e.*, incorporation into enamel, on the plaque, or surface adsorption, etc. The effects of elements, therefore, can be compared only when the form of administration is through equal routes.

**Time (Age) of Administration.** The time at which the element is given has a profound influence with regard to the development of the animal and the stage of development of the tooth. Certain elements may exhibit toxic properties when fed to young immature animals and, therefore, inhibit their growth and development, the result being a sick and abnormal animal with unphysiological responses. The stage of development of the tooth is an even more important factor, for if the element is to be incorporated or adsorbed by the tooth, this can take place only at the initial stages of development or eruption and not when the enamel mineral has matured and lost its reactivity (*133*).

**Chemistry and Availability of the Mineral Compound.** The chemical structure, valence, and solubility are fundamental factors which also determine the activity of the element with regard to dental caries. The chemical properties of a compound being tested influence the intestinal absorption, the oral and intestinal flora, and the direct local uptake by the tooth or plaque. Experiments, therefore, even though they may use similar levels of a certain element, are not comparable if the chemical structure of the compound is different. Examples have been cited where a chemical form is effective at a particular tooth development stage and not at another later stage.

**Requirement and Toxicity Levels: Biological Reserves.** Trace elements play a part in many biological reactions, and some are definitely essential nutrients; no normal development can take place in their absence. The amounts required are usually extremely small, and it is very difficult to investigate the part played by such low concentrations of elements. It is not at all surprising, therefore, that uncertainty exists about the significance of some trace elements with regard to nutrition and dental health. Another problem that confronts the investigator is that all living matter contains trace elements, and they store them in organs such as the liver in vertebrates or other structures in the lower forms. The end result is that it is quite impossible to deplete the organism's biological reserves of nutrients enough to observe a clear dental effect or nutritional symptoms of a trace element deficiency.

The low requirements of these trace elements together with the high toxicity exhibited by many elements further complicates their investigations, for slightly higher levels usually bring about toxic effects which influence the physiological status and thereby obscure the interpretation of experiments, as is the case with selenium or molybdenum.

**Type of Diet.** In dental caries research, the type of diet used determines to a large extent the amount, type, and distribution of carious lesions in the molars. Nutritionally, diet determines the degree of well-being and normal development and maintenance of experimental animals, but in caries research, certain diets have built-in imbalances, mainly in the amounts of protein and minerals which are responsible for its cariogenicity. Caries-promoting diets, to be effective, have to allow the development of different types of lesions at the same time that they satisfy the requirements for normal development. Diets can be divided into natural, purified, and chemically defined (*130*). Work with trace elements requires the use of purified diets made up of a carbohydrate and protein source plus some oil and a salt and vitamin mixture. This type of diet has the advantage that its composition can be controlled and the trace elements can be kept constant, avoiding the fluctuations due to variations in the composition of plant food ingredients used in natural diets. Diet composition, feeding frequency, physical structure, and oral clearance are important factors in the conduct of experimental caries research.

**Interferences from Components of Diet.** The nature of the cariogenic diet influences the availability of trace elements from food materials, the storage of those elements in the tissues, their incorporation into their functional positions in the cell and, finally, their excretion. The metabolism of copper is markedly affected by molybdenum and that of molybdenum by the levels of inorganic sulfate in the diet. The zinc requirement apparently is increased when isolated soy-bean protein is used instead of casein as a protein source in purified diets. Phytic acid influences the uptake of calcium and iron in certain species, such as the pig.

Diets used in caries research should be studied carefully and screened out for possible interferences and mineral interactions which may bring about additional and unknown sources of variation in the experiments.

**Trace Elements or Contaminants.** The very low requirement of trace elements and the ubiquitous presence of trace elements in nature demand a rigid control of the environment surrounding experimental animals used in caries research. Trace element contaminants can come from the cage, especially if these are galvanized or have metal parts to which the animals have ready access; the water, if this is not carefully distilled and stored in tanks made of inert materials; diet ingredients; and the atmosphere, if air is not filtered and conditioned to proper temperature and humidity.

**Methods of Analysis and Caries Evaluation.** Trace element content of diets and water should be analyzed carefully in order to standardize the experimental conditions. Certain organs, besides teeth and other oral structures, should be dissected and analyzed for trace elements in order to understand their effects on the organism and, in particular, on the dental structures. The low levels of elements involved and the possibility of contamination during preparation of samples for analysis require the use of physical methods such as neutron activating analysis and electron probe microanalysis to understand their distribution in microstructures. Recently, the electron probe method of analysis has been greatly improved, enabling the researcher to scan a tooth structure and determine levels of elements such as P and Ca as well as lighter elements in 1-micron areas. In cases where this is not feasible, spectrographic analysis or the atomic absorption spectrophotometry become the methods of choice, for they are able to detect elements in parts per million levels. Large numbers of analyses can be carried out with the latter method, while the spectrographic procedure is useful in that several elements can be assayed readily in a sample.

The method used in the estimation of caries extent and severity is important, for it should be adequate for the type of lesion being formed by the cariogenic diet used and the duration of the experiment. Caries scoring methods differ in their reproducibility and in their specificities, and careful thought should be given to the choice of method and to the comparison of experimental results obtained in the different caries scoring procedures.

Other methods are used in caries research, such as hardness tests, solubility tests, dye penetration tests, etc., which are used to evaluate the effects of trace elements on tooth structure, but they all require a high degree of standardization in order to obtain meaningful and comparable results. These *in vitro* models should be cautiously evaluated, for they may be totally unrelated to the *in vivo* phenomena.

**Experimental Design.** A multiplicity of factors affect the results of dental caries experiments and interact between them, precluding the possibility of obtaining meaningful results from experiments where one of the factors is varied and the rest are maintained constant (*65, 98*).

Therefore, in the design of experiments in which many factors are involved, the so-called factorial experiment (*i.e.*, all combinations of all levels of all factors) or fractional factorials in which only some of the factors are statistically evaluated will allow estimates of existence of interactions. Factorial analysis has the disadvantage that as the number of factors increases, the experiment becomes extremely large. For instance, for 6 factors at only two levels, the factorial experiment requires $2^6 = 64$ trials. Statistical designs have been described for reducing the number of runs in large-scale fractional replication studies which enable the experimenter to draw up schedules which permit the examination of results at various stages of the research work. The selection of subsequent trials can be made as the results of the previous trials are obtained. Experimental designs of this type will make dental caries research experiments fruitful and effective.

### *Conclusion*

The results of an exhaustive literature review on the effect of trace elements in dental caries has been presented. Epidemiological data as well as experimental data obtained with animal studies indicate that the mineral portion of foods influences the prevalance of dental caries.

Trace elements may act as "bone-seeking" elements and accumulate in the skeleton and teeth to modify their development and composition as well as their chemical-physical properties. This influence, in the case of those elements in high concentration in surface enamel, may extend into the plaque, the oral flora, and the surrounding environment of the tooth.

When the literature is evaluated, a highly tentative classification can be made of the type of effect shown by trace elements with regard to dental caries, in spite of the fact that a large number of experiments present conflicting results. The source of confusion in these observations can be traced to the multiplicity of factors which enter into dental caries research and its relation to mineral nutrition.

Research work in which these factors are taken into consideration should be attempted in order to clarify the influence of mineral elements on dental caries.

### *Literature Cited*

(1) Adler, P., *Dent. Stomatol.* **1965,** 15, 96–110.
(2) Adler, P., *Odontol. Rev.* **1957,** 8, 52.
(3) Adler, P., Straub, J., *Acta Med. Acad. Sci. Hung.* **1953**, 4, 221–227.

(4) Andersen, C. A., Hasler, M. F., "X-Ray Optics and Microanalysis," p. 310, Herman, Paris, 1966.
(5) Anderson, R. J., *Brit. Dental J.* **1966**, 120, 271–275.
(6) Anderson, R. S., *Proc. ORCA Conf. Advan. Fluorine Res. and Dental Caries Prevent., 11th*, **1965**, 3, 165–169.
(7) Asgar, K., *J. Dental Res.* **1956**, 35, 742–748.
(8) Aslander, A., "Dental Caries: The Bone Meal Method and the Cariogenic Properties of Sugar," Royal Institute of Technology, Division of Agriculture, Stockholm, Sweden, 1960.
(9) Bachra, B. N., Trautz, O. R., Simon, O. L., *Arch. Oral Biol.* **1965**, 10, 731–738.
(10) Banks, S. O., Bhaskar, S. N., Weinmann, J. P., *Arch. Pathol.* **1951**, 51, 19–29.
(11) Battistone, G. C., Feldman, M. H., Reba, R. C., *Arch. Oral Biol.* **1967**, 12, 1115–1122.
(12) Baume, L. J., Mayer, J., *J. Dental Res.* **1966**, 45, 726–774.
(13) Becks, H., Furuta, W. J., *J. Am. Dental Assoc.* **1941**, 28, 1083–1088.
(14) Bibby, B. G., *J. Am. Med. Assoc.* **1961**, 177, 316–321.
(15) Bird, E. D., Thomas, W. C., *Proc. Soc. Exptl. Biol. Med.* **1963**, 112, 640–643.
(16) Birks, L. S., "Electron Probe Microanalysis," Wiley, New York, 1963.
(17) Bowen, W. H., *Arch. Oral Biol.* **1968**, 13, 713–714.
(18) Bowen, W. H., Eastoe, J. E., *Caries Res.* **1967**, 1, 130–136.
(19) Boyde, A., Switsur, V. R., Fearnhead, R. S., *J. Ultrastruct. Res.* **1961**, 5, 201–207.
(20) Boyers, C. L., Shaw, J. H., Rosenthal, E., Giordana, R., *J. Dental Res.* **1963**, 42, 1517.
(21) Brekhus, P. J., Armstrong, W. D., *J. Am. Dental Assoc.* **1936**, 23, 1459–1470.
(22) Briner, W. W., Rosen, S., *Arch. Oral Biol.* **1967**, 12, 1077–1084.
(23) Briner, W. W., Rosen, S., *Calcified Tissue Res.* **1968**, 2, 60–66.
(24) Brudevold, F., "The Chemistry and Prevention of Dental Caries," p. 32, R. F. Sognnase, Ed., C. C. Thomas, Springfield, Ill., 1962.
(25) Brudevold, F., Messer, A. C., *J. Dental Res.* **1961**, 40, 728 (Abstr.).
(26) Brudevold, F., Steadman, L. T., *J. Dental Res.* **1955**, 34, 209–216.
(27) *Ibid.*, **1956**, 35, 430–437.
(28) *Ibid.*, **1956**, 35, 749–752
(29) Brudevold, F., Steadman, L. T., Gardner, D. E., Rowley, J., Little, M. F., *J. Am. Dental Assoc.* **1956**, 53, 159–164.
(30) Brudevold, F., Steadman, L. T., Smith, F. A., *Ann. N. Y. Acad. Sci.* **1960**, 85, 110–132.
(31) Brudevold, F., Steadman, L. T., Spinelli, M. A., Amdur, B. H., Gron, P., *Arch. Oral Biol.* **1963**, 8, 135–144.
(32) Bryant, F. J., Henderson, E. H., Holgate, W., *Brit. Dental J.* **1960**, 108, 291–294.
(33) Butler, F. E., *Nature* **1961**, 189, 848–849.
(34) Buttner, W., *Advan. Fluorine Res. Dental Caries Prevent.* **1965**, 3, 19–30.
(35) Buttner, W., *Arch. Oral Biol. Spec. Suppl.* **1961**, 6, 40–49.
(36) Buttner, W., *J. Dental Res.* **1963**, 42, 453–460.
(37) Cadell, P. B., Cousins, F. B., *Nature* **1960**, 185, 863–864.
(38) Calonius, P. E. B., Visapaa, A., *Arch. Oral Biol.* **1965**, 10, 9–13.
(39) Campbell, W. J., Brown, J. D., *Anal. Chem.* **1968**, 40, 346R–375R.
(40) Claycomb, C. K., Sorenson, F. M., Gatewood, D. C., Jump, E. B., Weaver, M. E., *J. Dental Res.* **1961**, 40, 504–510.

(41) Claycomb, C. K., Summers, G. W., Jump, E. B., *J. Dental Res.* **1965,** 44, 826.
(42) Constant, M. A., Phillips, P. H., Elvehjem, C. A., *J. Nutr.* **1952**, 46, 271.
(43) Constant, M. A., Sievert, H. W., Phillips, P. H., Elvehjem, C. A., *J. Nutr.* **1954,** 53, 17–27.
(44) *Ibid.,* **1954,** 53, 29–41.
(45) Crane, D. B., *J. Dental Res.* **1960,** 39, 704.
(46) Cruickshank, D. B., *Biochem. J.* **1949,** 44, 299.
(47) Cruickshank, D. B., *Brit. Dental J.* **1940,** 68, 257–271.
(48) Dale, P. P., Keyes, P. H., *J. Dental Res.* **1945,** 24, 194.
(49) Dale, P. P., Powell, V. H., *J. Dental Res.* **1943**, 22, 33.
(50) Deakins, M., *J. Dental Res.* **1942,** 21, 429–435.
(51) Dreizen, S., Niedermeier, W., Dreizen, J. G., Spies, T. D., *J. Dental Res.* **1958,** 37, 1149–1156.
(52) Dreizen, S., Spies, H. A., Jr., Spies, T. D., *J. Dental Res.* **1952,** 31, 137–142.
(53) El Tannir, M. D., *Am. J. Public Health* **1959,** 49, 45.
(54) English, J. A., *J. Dental Res.* **1949,** 28, 172–194.
(55) Ericcson, Y., *Acta Odontol. Scand.* **1954,** 11, 167.
(56) Forbes, J. C., Smith, J. D., *J. Dental Res.* **1952,** 31, 129.
(57) Francis, M. D., Briner, W. W., *Arch. Oral Biol.* **1966,** 11, 349–354.
(58) Frank, R. M., Capitant, M., Goni, J., *J. Dental Res.* **1966,** 45, 672-682.
(59) Frazier, P. D., *Arch. Oral Biol.* **1967,** 12, 25–33.
(60) Geyer, C. F., *J. Dental Res.* **1953,** 32, 590–595.
(61) Ginn, J. T., Volker, J. F., *Proc. Soc. Exptl. Biol. Med.* **1944,** 57, 189.
(62) Gish, C. W., Muhler, J. C., Howell, C. L., *J. Dental Res.* **1957,** 36, 780.
(63) Goldenberg, H., Sobel, A. E., *Proc. Soc. Exptl. Biol. Med.* **1952,** 81, 695–698.
(64) Gustafson, G., Stelling, E., Brunius, E., *Acta Odontol. Scand.* **1963,** 21, 297–308.
(65) Guzman, M. A., "The Art and Science of Dental Caries Research," p. 131–149, Academic, New York, 1968.
(66) Hadjimarkos, D. M., *Brit. Dental J.* **1967,** 123, 201–202.
(67) Hadjimarkos, D. M., *Experientia* **1967,** 23, 930–932.
(68) Hadjimarkos, D. M., Bonhorst, C. W., *J. Pediat.* **1958,** 52, 274–278.
(69) Hadjimarkos, D. M., Bonhorst, C. W., *Nature* **1962,** 193, 177–178.
(70) Hadjimarkos, D. M., Bonhorst, C. W., *Oral Surg. Oral Med. Oral Pathol.* **1959,** 12, 113–116.
(71) Hadjimarkos, D. M., Starvick, C. A., Remmert, L. F., *J. Pediat.* **1952,** 40, 451–455.
(72) Hardwick, J. L., "Caries Resistant Teeth," p. 222–237, Ciba Foundation Symp., 1965.
(73) Harris, R. S., Navia, J. M., *Ann. N.Y. Acad. Sci.* **1968,** 153, 240–257.
(74) Harris, R. S., Nizel, A. E., *Intern. Congr. Nutr., 4th,* **1957,** p. 195.
(75) Harris, R. S., Nizel, A. E., *J. Dental Res.* **1959,** 38, 1142–1147.
(76) Head, J., *J. Am. Med. Assoc.* **1912,** 59, 2118–2122.
(77) Hein, J. W., "Advances in Experimental Caries Research," p. 197–222, G. R. Sognnaes, Ed., Am. Assoc. Advan. Sci., Washington, D. C., 1955.
(78) Hein, J. W., *J. Dental Res.* **1953,** 32, 654.
(79) Hein, J. W., Quigley, G. A., Marcussen, H., *J. Dental Res.* **1958,** 37, 34.
(80) Hein, J. W., Shafer, W. C., *J. Dental Res.* **1951,** 30, 510.
(81) Hein, J. W., Wisotzky, S., *J. Dental Res.* **1955,** 34, 756.
(82) Hendershot, L. C., Forsaith, J., *J. Dental Res.* **1958,** 37, 32–33.
(83) Hendershot, L. C., Monselll, E., Forsaith, J., "Metal-Binding in Medicine," pp. 306–311, J. J. Seven and A. L. Johnson, Eds., Lippincott, Philadelphia, 1960.

(84) Herrmann, M., Rozeik, F., *Deut. Zahnaerztl. Z.* **1962,** 17, 880–885.
(85) Hewat, R. E. T., Eastcott, D. F., "Dental Caries in New Zealand," Medical Research Council of New Zealand Publication, 1955.
(86) Hoerman, K. C., Klima, J. E., Birks, L. S., Nagel, D. S., Ludwick, W. E., Lyon, H. W., *J. Am. Dental Assoc.* **1966,** 73, 1301–1305.
(87) Holgate, W., Mole, R. H., Vaughan, J., *Nature* **1958,** 182, 1294–1295.
(88) Irving, J. T., *J. Physiol.* **1940,** 99, 8–17.
(89) Issac, S., Brudevold, F., *J. Dental Res.* **1957,** 36, 753–758.
(90) Jenkins, G. N., *Brit. Dental J.* **1967,** 122, 435–441.
(91) *Ibid.,* **1967,** 122, 500–503.
(92) *Ibid.,* **1967,** 122, 545–550.
(93) Johansson, B., *J. Dental Res.* **1965,** 44, 64–70.
(94) Johansen, E., Hein, J. W., *J. Dental Res.* **1953,** 32, 703.
(95) Johnson, A. R., Singer, L., *Arch. Oral Biol.* **1967,** 12, 389–399.
(96) Keyes, P. H., *J. Dental Res.* **1956,** 35, 95–101.
(97) Kinkel, H. J., Cremer, H. D., *J. Dental Res.* **1960,** 39, 640.
(98) Konig, K. G., "The Art and Science of Dental Caries Research," pp. 201–230, Academic, New York, 1968.
(99) Kruger, B. J., *J. Dental Res.* **1966,** 45, 714–725.
(100) Kruger, B. J., Univ. Queensland Papers, Dept. of Dentistry **1959,** 1, 1–28.
(101) Landing, B. H., Lahey, W. K., Schubert, J., Spinanger, J., *J. Dental Res.* **1957,** 36, 750.
(102) Leicester, H. M., *J. Dental Res.* **1946,** 25, 337.
(103) Leicester, H. M., Thomassen, P. R., Nicholas, L. W., *J. Dental Res.* **1954,** 33, 670.
(104) Little, M. F., Brudevold, F., *J. Dental Res.* **1958,** 37, 991–1000.
(105) Lobene, R. R., Burnett, C. W., *J. Dental Res.* **1954,** 33, 487.
(106) Losee, F. F., *Am. Assoc. Adv. Sci., Publ. 81,* **1964,** 41–54.
(107) Ludwig, T. G., Healy, W. B., Losee, F. L., *Nature* **1960,** 186, 695–696.
(108) Ludwig, T. C., Malthus, R. S., Healy, W. B., *Nature* **1962,** 194, 456–458.
(106) Losee, F. L., *Am. Assoc. Adv. Sci., Publ. 81,* **1964,** 41–54.
8–11.
(110) Lundquist, C., *J. Dental Res.* **1951,** 30, 203.
(111) Malthus, R. S., Ludwig, T. G., Healy, W. B., *N.Z. Dental J.* **1964,** 60, 291–296.
(112) Maynard, E. A., Downs, W. L., Scott, J. K., *Federation Proc.* **1950,** 9, 338.
(113) McClure, F. J., *J. Dental Res.* **1948,** 27, 34–40.
(114) McClure, F. J., Arnold, F. A., *J. Dental Res.* **1941,** 20, 97.
(115) McClure, F. J., McCann, H. G., *Arch. Oral Biol.* **1960,** 2, 151–161.
(116) McDonald, J. B., "Chemistry and Prevention of Dental Caries," p. 89, R. F. Sognnaes, Ed., C. C. Thomas, Springfield, Ill., 1962.
(117) Meckel, A. H., *J. Dental Res.* **1962,** 41, 1104.
(118) Miller, C. D., *J. Nutr.* **1963,** 80, 217–222.
(119) Moxon, A. L., Rhian, M., *Physiol. Rev.* **1943,** 23, 305.
(120) Muhlemann, H. R., Konig, K. G., *Helv. Odontol. Acta* **1964,** 8, Suppl. 1, 79–81.
(121) Muhler, J. C., *J. Dental Res.* **1957,** 36, 787–794.
(122) Muhler, J. C., *J. Indiana Dental Assoc.* **1960,** 39, 42.
(123) Muhler, J. C., Bixer, D., Shafer, W. C., *Proc. Soc. Exptl. Biol. Med.* **1956,** 93, 328.
(124) Muhler, J. C., Day, H. G., *J. Am. Dental Assoc.* **1950,** 41, 528.
(125) Muhler, J. C., Day, H. G., *J. Nutr.* **1951,** 44, 413.
(126) Muhler, J. C., Shafer, W. C., *J. Dental Res.* **1957,** 36, 895–896.

(127) Muhler, J. C., Shafer, W. C., *Science* **1954,** 119, 687.
(128) Munch, J., *Odontol. Rev.* **1957,** 8, 52.
(129) Myrback, K., *Z. Physiol. Chem.* **1926,** 159, 1–21.
(130) Navia, J. M., "The Art and Science of Dental Caries Research," pp. 245–255, Academic, New York, 1968.
(131) Navia, J. M., Cagnone, L. D., Lopez, H., Harris, R. S., *Proc. Intern. Assoc. Dental Res., 46th,* **1968,** p. 128.
(132) Navia, J. M., Henry, C. H., Lopez, H., Harris, R. S., *Federation Proc.* **1967,** 26, 415.
(133) Navia, J. M., Lopez, H., Harris, R. S., *Arch. Oral Biol.* **1968,** 13, 779–786.
(134) Navia, J. M., Lopez, H., Harris, R. S., *J. Nutr.* **1969,** 97, 133–140.
(135) Navia, J. M., Menaker, L., Seltzer, J., Harris, R. S., *Federation Proc.* **1968,** 27, 676.
(136) Neuman, W. F., Neuman, M. W., "The Chemical Dynamics of Bone Mineral," University of Chicago Press, Chicago, Ill., 1958.
(137) Nixon, G. S., Livingstone, H. D., Smith, H., *Arch. Oral Biol.* **1966,** 11, 247–252.
(138) Nixon, G. S., Livingstone, H. D., Smith, H., *Caries Res.* **1967,** 1, 327–332.
(139) Nixon, G. S., Smith, H., *J. Dental Res.* **1960,** 39, 514–516.
(140) *Ibid.,* **1962,** 41, 1013–1016.
(141) Nizel, A. E., Bibby, B. G., *J. Am. Dental Assoc.* **1944,** 31, 1619–1626.
(142) Nizel, A. E., Harris, R. S., *Arch. Biochem.* **1950,** 26, 155–157.
(143) Nizel, A. E., Harris, R. S., *J. Dental Res.* **1955,** 34, 513–515.
(144) Nizel, A. E., Harris, R. S., *N. Eng. J. Med.* **1951,** 244, 361–362.
(145) Parizek, J., *J. Endocrinol.* **1957,** 15, 56.
(146) Parizek, J., *Nature* **1956,** 177, 1036.
(147) Parma, C., Danek, J., Hanusova, N., *Cs. Stomatol.* **1952,** 52, 150.
(148) Picard, J., Cartier, P., Carties, A., *C.R. Soc. Biol.* **1952,** 146, 1488–1491.
(149) Pigman, W., Cueto, H., Baugh, D., *J. Dental Res.* **1964,** 43, Suppl. No. 6, 1187–1195.
(150) Pindborg, E. V., Pindborg, J. J., Plum, C. M., *Acta Pharmacol. Toxicol.* **1946,** 2, 302.
(151) Pindborg, J. J., *Oral Surg., Oral Med., Oral Pathol.* **1953,** 6, 780.
(152) Powell, V. H., Dale, P. O., *J. Dental Res.* **1943,** 22, 257.
(153) Ritchie, D. B., *Nature* **1961,** 190, 456–458.
(154) Rosser, H., Boyde, A., Stewart, A. D. G., *Arch. Oral Biol.* **1967,** 12, 431–440.
(155) Rozeik, F., Cramer, H. D., Hannover, R., *Deut. Zahnaerztl. Z.* **1956,** 11, 1104–1109.
(156) Russell, A. L., *in* "Environmental Variables in Oral Disease," pp. 21–39, Am. Assoc. Advan. Sci., Washington, D. C., 1966.
(157) Russell, A. L., *J. Dental Res.* **1963,** 42, 233–244.
(158) Rygh, O., *Bull. Soc. Chem. Biol.* **1949,** 31, 1052.
(159) Rygh, O., *Den Norske Tannloegeforeningst Idenc.* **1950,** 60, 1–19.
(160) Rygh, O., *Research* **1949,** 2, 443.
(161) *Ibid.,* **1950,** 3, 193–194.
(162) Schwarz, K., Foltz, C. M., *J. Am. Chem. Soc.* **1957,** 79, 3292.
(163) Schwarz, K., *Cited in Nutr. Rev.* **1958,** 16, 149, 174.
(164) Schwarz, K., *Vitamins Hormones* **1962,** 20, 463–484.
(165) Scott, D. B., Kaplan, H., Wyckoff, R. W. O., *J. Dental Res.* **1949,** 28, 31–47.
(166) Scrimshaw, N. S., Taylor, C. E., Gordon, J. E., *Am. J. Med. Sci.* **1959,** 237, 367–403.
(167) Shaw, J. H., *N.Y. State Dental J.* **1950,** 16, 503.

(168) Shaw, J. H., Griffiths, D., *Arch. Oral Biol.* **1961,** 5, 301–327.
(169) Sherman, B. S., Sobel, A. E., *J. Dental Res.* **1965,** 44, 454.
(170) Smith, M. I., Westfall, B. B., *Public Health Repts.* **1937,** 52, 1375.
(171) Sognnaes, R. F., *J. Nutr.* **1949,** 39, 147–157.
(172) Sognnaes, R. F., Shaw, J. H., *J. Dental Res.* **1953,** 32, 685.
(173) Sognnaes, R. F., Shaw, J. H., *J. Nutr.* **1954,** 53, 195–206.
(174) Soremark, R., *Acta Radiol. Suppl.* **1960,** 190, 1.
(175) Soremark, R., Lundberg, M., *Acta Odontol. Scand.* **1964,** 22, 255.
(176) Soremark, R., Samsahl, K., *Arch. Oral Biol.* **1961,** 6, 275–283.
(177) Speirs, R. L., *Caries Res.* **1967,** 1, 15–31.
(178) Steadman, L. T., Brudevold, F., Smith, F. A., *J. Am. Dental Assoc.* **1958,** 57, 340.
(179) Steadman, L. T., Brudevold, F., Smith, F. A., Gardner, D. E., Little, M. F., *J. Dental Res.* **1959,** 33, 285–292.
(180) Stephan, R. M., Harris, M. R., *J. Dental Res.* **1953,** 32, 708.
(181) Stookey, G. K., Muhler, J. C., *J. Dental Res.* **1960,** 39, 671.
(182) Stookey, G. K., Roberts, R. A., Muhler, J. C., *Proc. Soc. Exptl. Biol.* **1962,** 109, 702–706.
(183) Stralfors, A., *Arch. Oral Biol.* **1966,** 11, 149–161.
(184) *Ibid.,* **1966,** 11, 323–328.
(185) *Ibid.,* **1966,** 11, 609–615.
(186) *Ibid.,* **1967,** 12, 1375–1385.
(187) Suga, S., Gustafson, G., *Arch. Oral Biol. Suppl.* **1962,** 223–244.
(188) Swift, P., *Brit. Dental J.* **1967,** 123, 326–327.
(189) Takuma, S., Katagiri, S., Ozasa, S., *J. Electron Microscopy* **1966,** 15, 86–89.
(190) Tank, G., Storvick, C. A., *J. Dental Res.* **1960,** 39, 473–488.
(191) Tempestini, O., Pappalardo, G., *Panminerva Med.* **1960,** 38, 344.
(192) Thomassen, P. R., Leicester, H. M., *J. Dental Res.* **1959,** 38, 670.
(193) *Ibid.,* **1964,** 13, 346–352.
(194) Tipton, I. H., Foland, W. D., Bobb, F. C., McCorble, W. C., Oak Ridge National Lab. USAEC Report **CF-53-8-4,** 1953.
(195) Torell, P., *Odontol. Tidsk.* **1956,** 64, 165–183.
(196) Toth, K., *Acta Med. Hung.* **1954,** 6, 493–500.
(197) Tousimis, A. J., *Am. J. Med. Electronics* **1966,** 5, 15–20.
(198) Tousimis, A. J., "X-Ray Optics and X-Ray Microanalysis," pp. 539–557, Academic, New York, 1963.
(199) Van Reen, R., Ostrom, C. H., Berzinskas, V. J., *Arch. Oral Biol.* **1962,** 7, 351–359.
(200) Van Reen, R., Ostrom, C. A., Berzinskas, V. J., *Helv. Odontol. Acta* **1967,** 11, 53–59.
(201) Venkataramanan, K., Krishnaswany, N., *Indian J. Med. Res.* **1949,** 37, 277.
(202) Von der Fehr, F., *Advan. Fluorine Res. Dental Caries Prevent.* **1965,** 3, 83–98.
(203) Wadhwani, T. K., *J. Indian Inst. Sci.* **1954,** 36, 64.
(204) Wentz, J., *J. Dental Res.* **1955,** 34, 735.
(205) Wessinger, G. D., Weinmann, J. P., *Am. J. Physiol.* **1943,** 139, 233–238.
(206) Wheatcroft, M. G., English, J. A., Schlack, C. A., *J. Dental Res.* **1951,** 30, 523.
(207) Widdowson, E. M., McCance, R. A., Spray, C. M., *Clin. Sci.* **1951,** 10, 113–118.
(208) Winiker, M., *Odontol. Rev.* **1957,** 8, 42.
(209) Wisotzky, J., Hein, J. W., *IADR Meeting, 34th,* **1956,** No. 36.
(210) Wisotzky, J., Hein, J. W., *J. Am. Dental Assoc.* **1958,** 57, 797.
(211) Wisotzky, J., Hein, J. W., *J. Dental Res.* **1955,** 34, 735.

(212) *Ibid.*, **1955,** 34, 768.
(213) Wynn, W., Haldi, J., *J. Nutr.* **1954,** 54, 285–290.
(214) Wynn, W., Haldi, J., Law, M. L., *J. Dental Res.* **1960,** 39, 153–157.
(215) Wynn, W., Haldi, J., Law, M. L., Bentley, K. D., *J. Dental Res.* **1958,** 37, 33.
(216) Yaeger, J. A., *J. Dental Res.* **1963,** 42, 1178–1182.
(217) Zipkin, I., "Art and Science of Dental Caries Research," pp. 29–41, Academic, New York, 1968.
(218) Zipkin, I., Piez, K. A., *J. Dental Res.* **1950,** 29, 498.

RECEIVED October 27, 1969. Contribution Number **1118** from the Department of Nutrition and Food Science, Massachusetts Institute of Technology, Cambridge, Mass.

# 10

# Application of Chemical Agents for the Control of Dental Caries

ROBERT C. CALDWELL

School of Dentistry, University of California, Los Angeles, Calif. 90024

JOE P. THOMAS

School of Dentistry, University of Alabama, Birmingham, Ala. 35233

*Vehicles for caries-preventive agents include dentrifices, mouthwashes, chewing gum, drinking water, cereals, flour, milk, table salt, tablets, and concentrated solutions which are applied by dentists. Many chemicals reduce dental caries in experimental animals. Those which have been subjected to clinical trials on humans include NaF, $SnF_2$, $Na_2PO_3F$, and other fluorides; $CaHPO_4$, anionic detergents, antibiotics, chlorophyll, urea, and vitamins. As a group, the fluorides have been most effective, and no single procedure has yet been as effective at the public health level as water fluoridation. However, several new approaches have promise. For example, topical application of acidulated sodium or stannous fluoride solutions once a year has resulted in a substantial reduction in caries, and fluoride mouthwashes prevent caries more effectively than dentifrices.*

Many approaches have been developed to reduce dental caries by chemical means; however, even the most effective procedures cannot yet be expected to eradicate the disease. A complete program of dental caries prevention includes dietary management, good oral hygiene, patient education and motivation, and early treatment of initial carious lesions, as well as the utilization of the various chemical agents. The use of a therapeutic agent is, in some instances, part of the oral hygiene technique, while in other cases it may be in the form of a dietary supplement. Very large caries reductions are possible in individuals who receive complete preventive care, but the 55–65% reduction resulting from water fluoridation remains the best protection available at the public health level at this time.

The most effective regime for the chemical prevention of dental caries probably consists of a combination of procedures, including water fluoridation or some other means of fluoride ingestion during childhood, periodic application of a caries-preventive agent in a relatively high concentration to the tooth enamel surface, and regular application of a less concentrated booster preparation of the caries-preventive agent. The time interval recommended for the application of the concentrated agent varies somewhat depending on the agent being discussed, while the less concentrated booster agent is for more frequent use to maintain the chemical at or in the enamel surface between concentrated applications.

Caries-preventive chemical agents can be incorporated into a variety of vehicles which can be divided into four main categories.

(1) Agents applied by the dental team: These include concentrated solutions of various fluorides for topical application, prophylaxis pastes containing fluoride, various fluoride gels, and agents applied to inhibit the growth of dental bacterial plaque.

(2) Therapeutic agents prescribed for personal application: These include fluoride tablets, lozenges, drops, mouthwashes, prophylaxis pastes.

(3) Public health measures: These include water fluoridation, large scale supervised self-application of fluoride-containing agents, and the use of milk, table salt, bread, breakfast cereals, and flour as vehicles for fluoride or other caries-preventive agents such as certain phosphates.

(4) Over-the-counter preparations: These include dentifrices, mouthwashes, and chewing gum.

### *Agents Applied by Dental Team*

The current status of topical fluoride solutions has been reviewed by Horowitz and Heifetz (*45*). In general, there appears to be merit in the use of topical solutions and prophylaxis pastes containing fluoride for the reduction of dental caries; however, in spite of 25 years of clinical investigations into various solutions and techniques, no clearly superior solution or technique to date has been identified. Clinical testing methods today are relatively unrefined when compared with methods available in the physical sciences. Treatment effects, therefore, can be only estimated grossly. De Paola has appropriately commented that independent tests of the same or similar agents "frequently show marked differences in the percentages of reduction in dental caries; therefore, we should not take percentage reduction figures too literally, and reductions from one study to another should be compared with caution" (*16*).

The well-known method of topical application of sodium fluoride to the enamel surface described first by Bibby (*7*) has been widely used.

The procedure was developed by Knutson and coworkers (*30, 31, 54, 56–59*), who used a 2% sodium fluoride solution which was allowed to dry on the teeth for 3 to 5 minutes. The 2% sodium fluoride is applied at 4 weekly intervals with a prophylaxis being done at the first appointment only. This series of applications is repeated at age 3, 7, 11, and 13. These investigators reported reductions in dental caries (DFT) of 39.7, 41.4, and 36.7% after 1, 2, and 3 years, respectively. The majority of studies using this technique have shown dental caries incidence to be reduced 30 to 40% in the permanent teeth of children residing in an area with fluoride-deficient water. The major disadvantage of this thoroughly studied technique has been the necessity of four patient visits over a short period of time.

With the advent of stannous fluoride, many dentists switched to the technique of Muhler (*78*). The recommended procedure involves thorough initial prophylaxis and interproximal flossing and the application of a fresh 8% solution of stannous fluoride, keeping the teeth moist with the solution for 4 minutes. This technique has the advantage of involving a single visit for the initial treatment. It requires reapplication in 6 months to a year, depending on the individual caries susceptibility of the patient. Horowitz and Heifetz (*45*) summarized the extensive clinical investigations of stannous fluoride solutions by Muhler and his associates, who have reported a range of benefit of 47 to 78% reduction in DMF surfaces in children. This range of benefit is also assessed by Stookey (*51*) at from 40 to 60%, which is in excess of the range of benefit reported for the 2% NaF technique. A few studies have shown negative results with stannous fluoride (*47, 104, 113*), and disadvantages of taste, gingival blanching, instability of aqueous solutions, and unesthetic pigmentations have been pointed out (*51*).

Acidulated phosphate fluoride has been reviewed by De Paola (*16*). This relatively new agent consists of a solution of sodium fluoride adjusted to pH 3 by the addition of 0.1 *M* phosphoric acid. The solution contains 1.23% sodium fluoride and, in initial clinical studies, seemed to surpass agents already in use (*11, 81, 112*). Table I includes representative data showing that at the end of a two-year study a reduction in dental caries (DMFS) of 70% (*112*) resulted. Wellock, Maitland, and Brudevold, in an investigation (*113*) in which half the mouth was treated with 2% NaF and half with acidulated phosphate fluoride (APF), reported 50% fewer new carious lesions on the APF side of the mouth. This technique was also more successful with subjects who maintained good oral hygiene. The addition of acid to stannous fluoride was studied by Muhler, Stookey, and Bixler (*86*) with good results reported. Table I shows that Mercer and Muhler (*74*) and Scola and Ostrum (*97*) reduced the 4-minute stannous fluoride treatment to 15 or 30 seconds with no

**Table I. Recent Developments**

| *Principal Investigator* | *Age Group, Years* | *Solution Used* |
|---|---|---|
| | | *Acid Phosphate–* |
| Wellock (*112*) | 8–11 | 1.23% NaF in 0.1 *M* phosphoric acid |
| Pameijer (*87*) | 4–10 | 2% NaF in 0.15 *M* phosphoric acid |
| Muhler (*86*) | Grade School | 10% $NaH_2PO_4$ plus 8% $SnF_2$ |
| | | *15–30-Sec.* |
| Mercer (*74*) | 5–12 | 8% $SnF_2$ (4 min.)<br>10% $SnF_2$ (30 sec.) |
| Scola (*97*) | 17–24 | $SnF_2$ prophy paste, topical & dentifrice:<br>4 min. topical<br>15 sec. topical |
| Horowitz (*46*) | 7–9 | 8% $SnF_2$ 4 min. topical<br>10% $SnF_2$ 30 sec. topical |

apparent loss of effectiveness. However, in an evaluation of a 30-second application of a stannous fluoride solution, Horowitz and Heifetz (*46*) had disappointing results with this rapid technique. Averill *et al.* (*2*) in a 2-year study of the effects of three topical fluorides (2% aqueous sodium fluoride, 4% stannous fluoride, and 2% APF) applied twice annually in children living in a nonfluoridated community failed to show conclusive superiority of any one of these agents.

Caries-reducing chemical agents have been added to prophylaxis pastes. The addition of stannous fluoride and APF to prophylaxis pastes has been studied clinically. A caries reduction of 34% (DMFS) with a stannous fluoride prophylaxis paste was reported by Bixler and Muhler (*9*), while Gish and Muhler (*34*) have obtained about a 40% reduction (DMFS) with the same paste. In this study, the combined use of stannous fluoride paste and topical stannous fluoride was more effective than paste alone. Scola and Ostrum (*97*) reported a caries reduction of 12% after the use of a stannous fluoride prophylaxis paste, which is probably not a significant reduction; however, the paste seemed to enhance the effect of a topical solution and a stannous fluoride dentifrice.

Horowitz and Lucye (*48*) in a 2-year study of children receiving annual prophylaxis with the stannous fluoride–lava pumice paste observed no protection against caries incidence as compared to controls. Peterson and others (*89*) studied an acidulated fluoride–lava pumice prophylaxis paste applied annually in children in communities with fluoridated and others with nonfluoridated water supplies, and reported minimal reduction in dental caries increments.

Horowitz (*42–44*) studied the caries-reducing effect of an APF gel and solution. After 3 years, those receiving annual application of the

**in Topical Fluoride Therapy**

| *Frequency of Application* | *No. in Exptl. Group* | *Length of Study, Years* | *Caries Reduction (DMFS)* |
|---|---|---|---|
| *Fluoride* | | | |
| 1 per year | 115 | 2 | 70 |
| 4 × in 2 weeks | 77 | 15 mo. | 50[a] |
| 1 application | 100 | 9 mo. | 75 |
| *Application* | | | |
| 2 per year | 135 | 2 | 56 |
| 2 per year | 132 | 2 | 59 |
| 1 per year | 200 | 1 | 45 |
| 1 per year | 194 | 1 | 54 |
| 1 per year | 420 | 3 | 21 |
| 1 per year | 421 | 3 | 3.8 |

[a] Compared to effect of 2% NaF.

APF solution experienced a 24% reduction in dental caries (DMFS) while those receiving semiannual application of the APF solution had a 41% reduction in caries incidence. The APF gel was applied in a wax tray and produced a 21% reduction as compared with the controls. Ingraham and Williams (*52*) evaluated an APF gel and solution. After 2 years, those treated with the gel demonstrated a 41% effect as compared with controls. Beneficial results from treatment with the APF solution were minimal. Bryan and Williams (*12*) reported a 28% dental caries reduction after 1 year using an APF gel in a foam rubber tray in one application. One report showed no effect as compared with controls of 1 application of APF gel (*102*). Cons, Janerich, and Senning (*15*), in a 3-year study to evaluate the caries-preventive effect of four topical fluoride procedures as compared with controls, found that, statistically, the group treated with APF gel experienced significantly fewer new carious teeth than the control group but the actual difference was small. The agents studied were sodium fluoride, 2%; stannous fluoride, 8%; APF fluoride solution, 1.23% at pH 3; and an APF fluoride gel, also 1.23% at pH 3. The treatments were given annually. The difference between the other treatments and the controls was not statistically significant. The technique for applying chemical by the use of an applicator tray or mouthpiece which holds the active agent against the enamel surface was reported by Horii and Keyes (*41*).

Stralfors (*99*) has described a "disinfectant cap splint" containing a thin layer of a fine-grained powdered disinfectant such as Chloramine-T. The splint containing the disinfectant is worn over the teeth for 5 minutes, and Stralfors reported an almost 100% decrease in the number of surviving bacteria. After about 6 hours the bacterial count rises, and by 12 hours has almost reached the original level.

### *Therapeutic Agents Prescribed for Personal Application*

In areas where the water is deficient in fluoride supplements, various other forms of fluoride have been prescribed for systemic use. A brief discussion of certain aspects of systemic fluoride therapy follows. For more extensive information, the review of Birch (*8*) is recommended.

Tablets usually contain 2.21 mg of sodium fluoride (1 mg $F^-$), which is equivalent to the average amount of fluoride ingested daily from water which contains 1 ppm fluoride. Apart from Arnold, McClure, and White's study (*1*) in which the beneficial effect of fluoride tablets was equated with that of fluoridated water, most studies indicate fluoride tablets to be no more than half as effective in reducing dental caries as fluoridated water. Birch states in his review that the reduction in dental caries incidence in eight studies ranged from 12 to 87% but that the use of fluoride in tablets to reduce caries incidence remains to be proved factually in long-term clinical investigation. The use of fluoride in tablets appears to have great potential but requires further study.

Multiple vitamin–fluoride tablets have been prescribed by physicians and dentists. Hennon, Stookey, and Muhler (*39*) in 1967 reported on an investigation of the effect of the daily use of fluoride vitamins by infants and by children up to 5 years of age. After 48 months, a reduction in the prevalence of carious lesions of 68% (def surfaces) in primary and 46% (DMF surfaces)in permanent teeth had resulted. Doherty (*17*) reviewed the use of dietary fluorides and does not encourage the use of vitamin–fluorides because of the need to adjust the dose with varying water fluoride content and the need for further study on the effect on permanent teeth. Also, the Committee on Nutrition of the American Academy ot Pediatrics questions the routine administration of vitamin supplements.

Fluoride passes through the placenta and is deposited in the bones and teeth of the developing child. There seems to be a regulatory mechanism involved which limits the amount cf fluoride transferred because even in areas of endemic fluorosis one does not see mottling of primary teeth. The effect of prenatal exposure to fluoridation has been reviewed by Horowitz and Heifetz (*47*), who reported no meaningful benefits to be derived from dietary supplements of fluoride to pregnant women. The Food and Drug Administration in its "Statements of general policy or interpretation, oral prenatal drugs containing fluorides for human use" (*29*), banned marketing by manufacturers of dietary supplements of fluoride offered to gravid women for "prenatal decay prevention."

Various U.S. pharmaceutical companies apparently do not adhere to the dosage schedule recommended by the American Council on Dental Therapeutics. The dosages suggested on the labels of different manufacturers of fluoride tablets and drops vary, as do the instructions as to when or when not to use systemic fluoride therapy. It is not surprising that there should be some confusion about fluoride prescriptions because there are over 40 different kinds of fluoride tablets, lozenges, or drops on the U.S. market.

Fluoride mouthwashes will be discussed along with other mouthwashes in the section on over-the-counter preparations.

### *Public Health Measures*

It has been established beyond any reasonable doubt that water fluoridation is a highly desirable and effective public health measure. In this country, the state legislature of Connecticut led the way in making fluoridation available on a state-wide basis, and now Minnesota, Illinois, Delaware, Michigan, South Dakota, and Ohio require fluoridation of public water supplies. Several other states are considering similar legislation. In Ireland, fluoridation has been approved for the entire country. Hopefully, these actions foretell a national fluoridation act for the United States. Knutson (*55*) estimated that 70% of the U.S. population now has access to water fluoridation. In areas where the water does not contain enough fluoride, a number of other methods have been employed to make fluoride available on a public health level.

### *Supervised Self-Application of Fluoride Agents*

The idea of large numbers of children in school applying fluoride to their own teeth apparently originated in Sweden. Berggren and Welander (*5*) evaluated a 1% solution of sodium fluoride which 568 children brushed on their teeth nine times over a 2-year period, achieving a 25–30% reduction in caries on the upper teeth. In the past few years, several other studies have been published in which a variety of solutions have been used (Table II). Sodium fluoride also has been used as a 0.5% solution or as 1.23% sodium fluoride in 0.1 *M* phosphoric acid. In the case of the weaker solution, used five times a year, there was a 29% reduction in caries (DMFT) (*6*). The acidulated 1.23% sodium fluoride used five times a year resulted in a 15% caries reduction (DMFS) (*13*). Goaz *et al.* (*37*) observed an additional 42% caries reduction in a city with fluoridated water by daily brushing with 6% sodium monofluorophosphate. After 21 months, Goaz *et al.* (*36*), using a caries index not in common use and having a number of reversals in diagnosis, reported a

**Table II. Caries Reduction with Fluoride**

| *Principal Investigator* | *Age Group, Years* | *Solution Used* | *Frequency of Application* |
|---|---|---|---|
| Berggren (*5*) | 8–15 | 1% NaF | 5 × 1st yr., 4 × 2nd yr. |
| Rosenkranz (*94*) | 12–14 | Zirconium–citrate–fluoride (0.42% NaF) | 6/year |
| Goaz (*37*) | 6–14 | 6% Sodium monofluorophosphate | 1/day Unsupervised |
| Berggren (*6*) | 10 | 0.5% NaF | 5/year |
| | | | 2/year |
| | | Zirconium fluoride | 5/year |
| | | (0.11% $F^-$) | 2/year |
| | | Ferric fluoride | 5/year |
| | | (0.36% $F^-$) | 2/year |
| Hunstadbraten (*50*) | 7–14 | 1% NaF | 4/year |
| Bullen (*13*) | 6–8 | 1.23% NaF in 0.1 *M* phosphoric acid | 4–5/year |

50% reduction in rate of decay. A large-scale program among the military was reported by Kyes (*62*), which consisted of supervised tooth brushing by the patient with an 8% stannous fluoride–lava pumice paste, application of 10% stannous fluoride solution for 15 seconds or more, and the use of a stannous fluoride dentifrice. Scola (*96*) reported a 50% reduction in increment of dental caries as compared to controls in this military program after 1 year. Other studies have been reported regarding the use of self-administered stannous fluoride–zirconium silicate prophylactic paste (*73, 76, 81*). It was estimated (*92*) that in 1969 over 1,500,000 applications by this method would be occurring. Lang *et al.* (*64*) reported results of four applications at 6-month intervals of a 9% stannous fluoride–zirconium silicate prophylaxis paste which also contained 9% monosodium dihydrogen phosphate. A reduction in dental caries increment (DMFS) of about 40% was noted. The children studied resided in a fluoridated community. The addition of a stannous fluoride dentifrice resulted in no significant further decrease in caries increments.

Englander and others (*24*), using a custom-fitted upper and lower mouthpiece, studied repeated application of acidulated and neutral water-soluble sodium fluoride gels for 21 months. One group applied an acidulated phosphate sodium fluoride gel 6 minutes each school day for 2 academic years and the second group followed the same procedure with the neutral sodium fluoride gel. A third group served as control. After 21 months, outstanding results of 75 and 80% reduction in dental caries increment (DMF surfaces) occurred with the two groups as compared

**Solutions Brushed on the Teeth**

| *No. in Exptl. Group* | *Length of Study, Years* | *Per Cent Caries Reduction (DMFS)* | *Comments* |
|---|---|---|---|
| 568 | 2 | 25–30 | More effective on upper teeth than on lower |
| 84 | 1 | 34 | |
| 96 | 14 mo. | 42 | Drinking water fluoridated (1 ppm) for 10 yr |
| 177 | 2 | 29[a] | |
| 174 | 2 | 17[a] | |
| 176 | 2 | 17[a] | |
| 162 | 2 | 0[a] | |
| 167 | 2 | 33[a] | |
| 170 | 2 | 8[a] | |
| 800 | 2 | | "Significant reduction" |
| 235 | 2 | 15 | |

[a] DMFT values.

with controls (*23*). Recently, the authors reported that 23 months after the treatments had been discontinued, the children available for reexamination still retained the advantage of 55 and 63% fewer new DMF surfaces than the control children. In the study, the higher percentage effect was obtained with the acidulated fluoride gel. Muhler *et al.* (*82*) reported on the clinical evaluation of patient-administered stannous fluoride zirconium silicate prophylactic paste in children in the Virgin Islands. After one year, children using the treatment paste containing 9% stannous fluoride obtained a reduction in new DMF surfaces of 64% as compared with children applying a prophylaxis paste containing no fluoride.

### *Fluoridation of the Diet*

Until all the water supplies which can be fluoridated economically in this country have been supplemented with fluoride, fluoridation of the diet will be of secondary importance to most public health groups. However, even when all of the available water supplies have been fluoridated, a very large number of citizens in rural areas and in small towns still will not have the benefits of fluoride unless some method other than water fluoridation is devised. Accordingly, some of the studies which have been conducted in Europe adding fluoride to the daily diet of children are of considerable importance. Table salt has been fluoridated in some

**Table III. Reduction in Dental Caries**

| *Principal Investigator* | *Age Group, Years* | *Length of Study, Years* | *Number in Exptl. Group* |
|---|---|---|---|
| Muhler (*84*) | 5–15 | 1 | 214 |
| Muhler (*85*) | 5–15 | 1 | 219 |
| Muhler (*83*) | 17–36 | 2 | 131 |
| Muhler (*79*) | 6–15 | 1 | 257 |
| Jordan (*53*) | 8–11 | 2 | 190 |
| | | | 104 |
| Muhler (*80*) | 6–18 | 2 | 189 |
| Peffley (*88*) | 10–19 | 10 mo. | 156 |
| Hill (*40*) | 9–16 | 2 | 189 |
| Kyes (*63*) | 17–24 | 2 | 180 |
| Muhler (*75,77*) | 6–18 | 3 | 165 |
| Bixler (*9*) | 6–17 | 1 | 219 |
| | | | 230 |
| Zacherl (*114*) | 6–7 | 1.5 | 461 |
| | 12 | 1.5 | 408 |
| Gish (*34*) | 6–14 | 1 | 206 |
| Gish (*35*) | 6–14 | 1 | 207 |
| Torell (*105*) | 10 | 2 | 169 |
| Held (*38*) | 13–17 | 4 | 66 |
| Thomas (*103*) | 7–16 | 2 | 158 |
| Horowitz (*49*) | 6–10 | 3 | 288 |

parts of Switzerland, resulting in a reduction in dental caries. In discussing these Swiss findings, Ericsson (*25*) pointed out that too little fluoride was added to the salt and that a substantial effect on the incidence of dental caries is possible with the correct formulation. It is generally considered that the distribution problem in the U.S. would be too great to make fluoridated table salt a practical dental public health measure.

Fluoridation of milk is a logical idea because the distribution of school milk is already in effect in many areas. Fluoride is compatible with milk and in the study by Rossoff *et al.* (*95*) in Louisiana, 1 mg fluoride ion as sodium fluoride was added by 6–10 year old children to the half pint of milk consumed daily. After 3½ years, it appeared that caries was reduced by 70% in newly erupted permanent teeth as compared with teeth of controls. This investigation and others reviewed by Birch (*8*) point out the need for further study of the effectiveness of dietary supplement with fluoride in milk.

The addition of caries-preventive chemicals to flour used for bread or baked goods has been the subject of studies in several countries. Flour used for bread baking is often enriched by $CaHPO_4$ or $CaCO_3$ to provide

**with Stannous Fluoride Dentrifices**

| Per Cent Caries Reduction (DMFS) | | | |
|---|---|---|---|
| *1 yr.* | *2 yr.* | *3 yr.* | *Comments* |
| 49 | – | – | |
| 36 | – | – | |
| 41 | 34 | – | |
| 23 | – | – | |
| 34 | 21 | – | Supervised brushing once daily |
| – | 12 | – | |
| 23 | 25 | – | |
| 57 | – | – | Supervised brushing 3 × daily |
| 14 | 15 | – | |
| 1 | 14 | – | |
| 19 | 19 | 22 | |
| 1[a] | – | – | Plus $SnF_2$ prophylaxis paste |
| 40[a] | – | – | Plus $SnF_2$ paste and topical |
| 39 | 42 | – | 10 and 18 month results |
| 34 | 39 | – | 10 and 18 month results |
| 7[a] | – | – | Plus $SnF_2$ paste and topical |
| 35[a] | – | – | 0.91 ppm fluoride in water |
| – | 21[a] | – | |
| Significant reduction | | | Supervised brushing 2 × daily with NaF–$SnF_2$ dentifrice |
| 17 | 30(DFS) | – | Supervised brushing 3 × daily |
| 10 | 12 | 21 | Brushing at home and school |

[a] Calculated from authors' data.

a dietary calcium. With the comprehensive evidence available for a caries-protective effect of various phosphates in experimental animals, Stralfors (*100*) incorporated 2% $CaHPO_4 \cdot 2H_2O$ into soft bread, hard bread, wheat flour used for cooking, and sugar in a 2-year study of 2102 children, half of whom ate the phosphate-enriched bread and half of whom ate the bread without phosphate. Although caries was inhibited by 50% in the experimental group the first year and 40% the second year, evaluation was difficult since the dicalcium phosphate used contained 250 ppm fluoride the first year and only 25 ppm fluoride the second year. This made separation of the phosphate effect impossible. Since Averill and Bibby (*3*) and Ship and Mickelsen (*98*) failed to find a significant caries reduction with 2% dicalcium phosphate incorporated into bread, pastries, desserts, or sugar, it seems that this approach to caries prevention requires further study. The use of phosphates as a diet supplement to effect dental caries activity has been reviewed by Gilmore (*33*).

The addition of fluoride to bread has been proposed from time to time. Ericsson (*25*) has reviewed the feasibility of this procedure and points out that in Holland there is less variation in bread consumption than in water consumption. Likewise, Ege (*20*) has shown that in Denmark the consumption of cereals varies less than drinking water. Therefore, in these two countries at least, the fluoridation of cereals seems feasible.

### *Over-the-Counter Preparations*

Despite all of the scientific and advertising furor, none of the dentifrices available at the present time is likely to reduce dental caries in children under conditions of home use by more than 25–30%. Less would be expected if adults used these products. Volker and Caldwell (*109*), Wallace (*110*), Mandel and Cagan (*68*), Bartelstone *et al.* (*4*), and Hill (*40*) have reviewed the early investigations of dentifrices containing therapeutic agents for dental caries reduction. For the purpose of this paper, stannous fluoride dentifrices will be reviewed and some recent developments with other agents will be discussed. Table III contains the pertinent data. The University of Indiana School of Dentistry and the Indiana Department of Public Health have been responsible for the majority of reports dealing with stannous fluoride dentifrices. Usually their results have been favorable, although two reports are difficult to evaluate. Bixler and Muhler (*9*) found no dentifrice effect after use of a stannous fluoride prophy paste but they observed a 40% dentifrice effect following stannous fluoride prophy paste and stannous fluoride topical. This contrasts with Gish and Muhler's (*34*) finding of little or no dentifrice effect with stannous fluoride prophy paste and stannous fluoride topical. Apart from favorable results from the many Indiana studies, Jordan and Peterson (*53*), Hill (*40*), Kyes, Overton, and McKean (*63*) have had negative results in studies of unsupervised brushing, while Torell and Ericsson (*105*) have obtained about a 25% reduction, Zacherl and McPhail (*114*) a 42% reduction, and Thomas and Jamison (*103*) a 30% reduction when the teeth were brushed three times daily. Held and Spirgi (*38*) in a study of a NaF–$SnF_2$ dentifrice also have observed a significant reduction in caries.

An interesting series of papers on fluoride dentifrice trials appeared in the *British Dental Journal* (*10*). Five studies were described, all involving stannous fluoride dentifrices. In some studies, the dentifrice abrasive was insoluble metaphosphate. In one of the studies, a sodium monofluorophosphate was also evaluated. These well planned and executed studies were carried out under rigorous conditions involving use of the double blind technique with adequate sample sizes followed long enough to demonstrate real differences between groups. Some general conclusions came out of the five studies. First, apparently the early problem of incompatibility between the abrasive in the dentifrice and the

**Table IV. Therapeutic Dentrifices for Dental Caries**

| *Type of Active Ingredient* | *Mechanism of Action* | *Chemical Agents Used* | *General Conclusions about Effectiveness* |
|---|---|---|---|
| Detergent | Antienzyme | Sodium dehydroacetate<br>Sodium lauroyl sarcosinate | Limited effect possible; variable results |
| Urea | Buffering, protein denaturation | Dibasic ammonium phosphate<br>Urea | Ineffective in the low concentrations used |
| Antibiotic | Antibacterial | Penicillin<br>Tyrothrycin | Doubtful if suitable for general use |
| Fluoride | Antienzyme, decreased enamel dissolution, increased remineralization | Amine fluoride<br>Sodium fluoride<br>Sodium monofluorophosphate<br>Stannous fluoride | Limited effect |
| Surface-coating agent | Reduced adhesion of food and bacteria to enamel | Tetradecylamine | Ineffective |

fluoride has been largely overcome, and stable products with active fluorides are now available. Second, in all five studies, stannous fluoride dentifrices caused staining of the teeth. In one report, the increase in staining was described as a tremendous increase in brown stain. This undesirable effect of stannous fluoride dentifrices indicates that non-tin-containing dentifrices seem to hold more promise for future study and use. A sodium monofluorophosphate dentifrice was slightly, although not significantly, more effective than stannous fluoride dentifrice and did not stain the teeth. In a previous study by Finn and Jamison (27) in the U.S., it was shown that monofluorophosphate was more effective than a stannous fluoride dentifrice. A third finding in the British studies was that girls benefitted more from the use of the therapeutic dentifrices than boys, probably because of their better oral hygiene habits. It is somewhat disappointing to observe that little improvement in oral hygiene had resulted at the end of a 3-year program of oral hygiene instruction and regular tooth brushing. The reduction in caries reported ranged from no reduction in caries to 36% reduction in proximal caries of posterior

**Table V. Reduction in Dental Caries**

| *Principal Investigator* | *Age Group, Years* | *Solution Used* |
|---|---|---|
| Weisz (*111*) | 5–6<br>8–9 | 0.25% NaF<br>0.25% NaF |
| Torell (*106*) | 8–9 | 0.2% NaF<br>0.2% KF |
| Lundstam (*67*) | 7–15 | 0.2% NaF |
| Torell (*105*) | 10 | 0.05% NaF<br>0.2% NaF |
| McCormick (*72*) | 6–8 | Ca, $PO_4$, $F^-$ (3 ppm)<br>$F^-$ (3 ppm)<br>$F^-$ (40 ppm) |

tooth surfaces. When the DMFS index was used, the reduction in caries was marginal. Only by making special computations on teeth which had erupted during the study could the observers detect any substantial effect of the fluoride dentifrice. These British studies tend to confirm the opinion concerning stannous fluoride dentifrices that they have a marginal effect in reducing dental caries. Duckworth (*19*) reviewed fluoride dentifrices, in particular trials in the United Kingdom, and concluded that dentifrices containing stannous fluoride had a small but useful role in the prevention of dental caries in teen-age school children. The greater benefits shown by girls demonstrated that prevention depends upon conscientious use.

Table IV summarizes in a very general way the current status of the various dentifrices which have been formulated to prevent dental caries. The most effective dentifrices contain fluoride in some form, but even these have a limited ability to protect against dental caries.

Some studies have been designed to provide a more stable dentifrice formulation by using either non-calcium-containing abrasives or fluorides other than stannous fluoride. Manly (*69*) and Ericsson (*24*) have drawn attention to the problem of tin and fluoride reacting with the abrasive, which, as mentioned earlier, was a problem with earlier stannous fluoride dentifrices. Dentifrices can vary widely in the compatibility of the ingredients, making it difficult to compare the effectiveness of different dentifrices or even the same dentifrice from time to time when slight modifications in the formula have been made.

An amine fluoride dentifrice has been developed in Switzerland (*71*), the rationale for the amine fluoride being that it has antienzyme action and is retained better on the enamel surface than other fluorides. Mar-

**with Fluoride Mouthwashes**

| *Frequency of Application* | *No. in Exptl. Group* | *Length of Study, Years* | *Per Cent Caries Reduction (DMFS)* |
|---|---|---|---|
| 2/day | 21 | 10 | 88 |
| 2/day | 11 | 4 | 87 |
| 1/month | 912 | 1 | Significant decrease in |
| 1/month | 520 | 1 | anterior proximal caries |
| 1/two weeks | 2400 | 9 mo. | 36 |
| 1/day | 160 | 2 | 49 |
| 1/two weeks | 172 | 2 | 21 |
| 1/day | 90 | 30 mo. | 45[a] |
| 1/day | 90 | 30 mo. | 0 |
| 1/day | 90 | 30 mo. | 23[a] |

[a] Reduction calculated for mesial surfaces of 6-year molar. No effect on occlusal surfaces.

thaler (*70*) reported caries inhibition after 7 years of unsupervised use of an amine dentifrice. The dentifrice containing the amine fluorides inhibited new carious lesions by 32% based on new DF surfaces. Less promising results were obtained by Ludwig (*66*) with a tetradecylamine dentifrice. The idea of reducing food and bacterial plaque retention on the tooth surface is logical, but so far no effective method has been devised for achieving this with a dentifrice.

It is amusing to notice in Held and Spirgi's (*38*) article that the name of one of the dentifrices tested was Drab—a name hardly likely to excite the U.S. advertising community.

Mouthwashes have been popular for centuries because of their refreshing properties and ability to mask mouth odor. However, not until recently have truly therapeutic mouthwashes been formulated to prevent dental caries. For several years, Weisz (*111*) has claimed that children in his practice have very high resistance to caries when an 0.25% NaF mouthwash is used twice daily. Table V summarizes some of the available studies on fluoride mouthwashes. It can be seen from Table V that fluoride mouthwashes offer definite possibilities for controlling dental caries. It is not known whether or not these benefits would be additional to other methods of caries control such as topical fluoride or fluoride pastes applied by the dentist, but it is quite possible that mouthwashes will prove to be more effective than dentifrices in reducing dental caries. The simple fact is that no incompatible or inactivating agents such as an abrasive or binder need be included in a mouthwash. An appraisal of Table V indicates that two factors influence the results, the frequency of mouthwashing and the strength of the fluoride solution. Although an editorial comment which accompanied one of Weisz's papers (*111*) suggested that an 0.25% NaF mouthwash is too concentrated for safe home use, as a practical matter, no problems seem to have been encountered by Weisz or other investigators. Certainly, the daily use of 0.05% NaF as studied by Torell and Ericsson (*105*) is very safe.

In comparing various procedures, Torell and Ericsson (*105*) found a daily mouthwash of 0.05% NaF was more effective than a 2% NaF mouthwash used once every 2 weeks. Likewise, the mouthwash was more effective than the standard techniques for topical 2% NaF or 10% $SnF_2$, or dentifrices containing stannous fluoride, or sodium monofluorophosphate. Fjaestad-Seger and others (*28*) reported that a weekly rinse with 0.2% neutral sodium fluoride or an iron fluoride solution showed a significant caries reduction in children. Torell and Sibert (*106*) studied monthly supervised rinsing of a 0.2% sodium fluoride solution among school children. As in the case of the other Swedish study (*28*), the effect was expressed as percentage of children receiving new restorations after one year. Using this less precise assessment, 13 to 27% fewer children received care after one year. Swerdloff and Shannon (*101*), studying the feasibility of the use of a stannous 0.4% fluoride mouthwash daily in a school preventive dentistry program, were able to report a 30.5% reduction in new carious surfaces after only 5 months. This time period and the small number of subjects studied made the results not significant other than to lend support to the other studies quoted.

A new development is the use of a "remineralizing" mouthwash. The rationale for this mouthwash is based on the evidence of Koulourides, Cueto, and Pigman (*60*) and Koulourides and Reed (*63*) that softened enamel can be rehardened by solutions of calcium and phosphorus and that the process is accelerated by small amounts of fluoride. McCormick and Koulourides (*72*) reported that the remineralizing mouthwash is capable of reducing caries on the mesial surface of the first molar by 45%.

The use of chewing gum as a vehicle for caries-preventive compounds predates several of the other methods described in this paper. A good review of the subject has been published by Richardson and Castaldi (*93*). Table VI summarizes the effect of chewing gum on dental caries. The first fact which should be mentioned is that in no published study have gum chewers had more caries than nonchewers. Actually, as shown by Dreizen and Spies (*18*), Volker (*108*), and Toto, Rapp, and O'Malley (*107*), ordinary chewing gum seems neither to cause nor prevent dental caries. Promising results by incorporating vitamin K, Furadoxyl (a nitrofuran), or chlorophyll in gum have been reported but none of these has been followed up. In a country such as the U.S.A., where chewing gum is widely used, this approach has untapped potential. It has been re-

**Table VI. Effect of Chewing Gum on Dental Caries**

| *Principal Investigator* | *Type of Gum Additive* | *Number in Exptl. Group* | *Type of Subjects* | *Duration of Study* | *Caries Reduction* |
|---|---|---|---|---|---|
| Burrill (*14*) | Synthetic vit. K | 55 | Dental students | 18 mo. | 60–90% |
| Dreizen (*18*) | Furadoxyl | 30 | Age 6–38 | 12 mo. | 80% |
| Gerke (*32*) | Chlorophyll | 102 | Adults (bakers) | 12 mo. | 20% (approx.) |
| Lind (*65*) | Potassium fluoride | 229 | Age 11 | 12 mo. | None |
| Burrill (*14*) | None | 45 | Dental students | 18 mo. | 13–80% |
| Volker (*108*) | None | 50 | Age 18–32 | 18 mo. | None |
| Dreizen (*18*) | None | 25 | Age 8–35 | 12 mo. | None |
| Toto (*107*) | None | 275 | Primary school | 12 mo. | None |

ported that fluoride or dicalcium phosphate can be released from a gum while chewing (*21, 90, 91*). In a clinical study of phosphate-containing chewing gum (*27*), Finn and Jamison demonstrated reduction of caries incidence in children after a 2-year period of 39.7 to 52.9% considering proximal surfaces of teeth only.

### *Literature Cited*


(1) Arnold, F. A., McClure, F. J., White, C. L., *Dental Progr.* **1960,** 1, 8.
(2) Averill, H. M., Averill, J. E., Ritz, A. G., Little, M. F., *Am. J. Public Health* **1967,** 57, 1627.
(3) Averill, H. M., Bibby, B. G., *J. Dental Res.* **1964,** 43, 1150.
(4) Bartelstone, H. J., Mandel, I. D., Chilton, N. W., *N. Y. Dental J.* **1962,** 28, 147.
(5) Berggren, H., Welander, E., *Acta Odontol. Scand.* **1960,** 18, 209.
(6) *Ibid.,* **1964,** 22, 401.
(7) Bibby, B. G., *Tufts Dental Outlook* **1942,** 15, 4.
(8) Birch, R. C., *J. Public Health Dentistry* **1969,** 29, 170.
(9) Bixler, D., Muhler, J. C., *J. Am. Dental Assoc.* **1964,** 68, 792.
(10) *Brit. Dental J.* **1967,** 123 (1).
(11) Brudevold, F., Gron, P., Spinelli, M., Trantz, O., *Arch. Oral Biol.* **1963,** 8, 167.
(12) Bryan, E. T., Williams, J. E., *J. Public Health Dentistry* **1968,** 28, 182.
(13) Bullen, D. C. T., McCombie, F., Hole, L. S., *J. Can. Dental Assoc.* **1966,** 32, 89.
(14) Burrill, D. Y., Calandra, J. C., Tilden, E. B., Fosdick, L. S., *J. Dental Res.* **1945,** 24, 273.
(15) Cons, N. C., Janerich, D. T., Senning, R. S., *J. Am. Dental Assoc.* **1970,** 80, 777.
(16) De Paola, P. F., *J. Am. Coll. Dentists* **1968,** 35, 22.
(17) Doherty, J. M., *Wis. Med. J.* **1968,** 67, 599.
(18) Dreizen, S., Spies, T. D., *J. Am. Dental Assoc.* **1951,** 43, 147.
(19) Duckworth, R., *Brit. Dental J.* **1968,** 124, 505.

(20) Ege, R., *Tandlaegebladet* **1961,** 65, 445.
(21) Emslie, R. D., Veall, N., Duckworth, R., *Brit. Dental J.* **1961,** 110, 121.
(22) Englander, H. R., Carlos, J. P., Senning, R. S., *et al., J. Am. Dental Assoc.* **1969,** 78, 783.
(23) Englander, H. R., Keyes, P. H., Gestwicki, M., Schultz, H. A., *J. Am. Dental Assoc.* **1967,** 75, 638.
(24) Ericsson, Y., *in* "Caries Symposium Zurich," H. Muhlemann, Ed., Hans Huber, Berne, 1961.
(25) Ericsson, Y., *in* "Nutrition and Caries Prevention," G. Blix, Ed., Almqvist and Wiksells, Uppsala, 1965.
(26) Finn, S. B., Jamison, H. C., *J. Dental Assoc.* **1967,** 74, 987.
(27) Finn, S. B., Jamison, H. C., *J. Dentistry Children* **1963,** 30, 17.
(28) Fjaestad-Seger, M., Norstedt-Larsson, K., Torell, P., *Sveriges Tandlakarforb Tindn* **1961,** 53, 169.
(29) Food and Drug Administration, *Federal Register* **1966,** Oct. 20.
(30) Galagan, D. J., Knutson, J. W., *Public Health Rept.* **1947,** 62, 1477.
(31) *Ibid.,* **1948,** 63, 1215.
(32) Gerke, J., Klimt, W., *Zahnnaerztl. Rundschau* **1955,** 64, 499.
(33) Gilmore, N. D., *J. Public Health Dentistry* **1969,** 29, 88.
(34) Gish, C. W., Muhler, J. C., *J. Am. Dental Assoc.* **1965,** 70, 914.
(35) Gish, C. W., Muhler, J. C., Stookey, G. K., *J. Am. Dental Assoc.* **1965,** 71, 60.
(36) Goaz, P. W., McElwaine, L. P., Biswell, H. A., *et al., J. Dental Res.* **1966,** 45, 286.
(37) Goaz, P. W., McElwaine, L. P., Biswell, H. A., White, W. E., *J. Dental Res.* **1963,** 42, 965.
(38) Held, A. J., Spirgi, M., *Schweiz. Montsschr. Zahnheilk.* **1965,** 75, 883.
(39) Hennon, D. K., Stookey, G. K., Muhler, J. C., *J. Dentistry Children* **1967,** 34, 439.
(40) Hill, T. J., *J. Am. Dental Assoc.* **1959,** 59, 1121.
(41) Horii, A. A., Keyes, P. H., *J. Dental Res.* **1964,** 43, 152.
(42) Horowitz, H. S., *IADR Program and Abstracts of Papers,* No. 549, March 1969.
(43) Horowitz, H. S., *J. Am. Dental Assoc.* **1969,** 78, 568.
(44) Horowitz, H. S., *J. Oral Therap.* **1968** (Jan.), 4, 286.
(45) Horowitz, H. S., Heifetz, S. B., *J. Am. Dental Assoc.* **1970,** 81, 166.
(46) Horowitz, H. S., Heifetz, S. B., *J. Dentistry Children* **1969,** 36, 355.
(47) Horowitz, H. S., Heifetz, S. B., *Public Health Rept.* **1967,** 82, 297.
(48) Horowitz, H. S., Lucye, H. S., *J. Oral Therap.* **1966** (July), 3, 17.
(49) Horowitz, H. S., Thompson, M. B., *J. Am. Dental Assoc.* **1967,** 74, 979.
(50) Hunsfadbraten, V. K., *Dent. Zahnaerztl. Z.* **1965,** 20, 336.
(51) "Improving dental practise through preventive measures," Ch. 5, p. 110, J. L. Bernier and J. C. Muhler, Eds., C. V. Mosby Co., St. Louis, 1966.
(52) Ingraham, R. Q., Williams, J. E., *J. Tenn. Dental Assoc.* **1970** (Jan.), 50, 5.
(53) Jordan, W. A., Peterson, J. K., *J. Am. Dental Assoc.* **1959,** 58, 42.
(54) Knutson, J. W., *J. Am. Dental Assoc.* **1948,** 36, 37.
(55) *Ibid.,* **1970,** 80, 765.
(56) Knutson, J. W., Armstrong, W. D., *Public Health Rept.* **1943,** 58, 1701.
(57) *Ibid.,* **1945,** 60, 1085.
(58) *Ibid.,* **1946,** 61, 1685.
(59) Knutson, J. W., Armstrong, W. D., Feldman, F. M., *Public Health Rept.* **1947,** 62, 425.
(60) Koulourides, T., Cueto, H., Pigman, W., *Nature* **1961,** 189, 226.
(61) Koulourides, T., Reed, J. L., *Arch. Oral Biol.* **1964,** 9, 585.
(62) Kyes, F. M., *J. Oral Therap.* **1967,** 3, 359.

(63) Kyes, F. M., Overton, N. J., McKean, T. W., *J. Am. Dental Assoc.* **1961,** 63, 189.
(64) Lang, L. H., Thomas, H. G., Taylor, J. A., Rothhaar, R. E., *J. Dentistry Children* **1970** (May-June), 37, 27.
(65) Lind, V., Stelling, E., Nystrom, S., *Odontol. Revy* **1961,** 12, 341.
(66) Ludwig, T. G., *N. Z. Dental J.* **1963,** 59, 220.
(67) Lundstam, R., *Sveriges Tandlakarforbund Tidn* **1964,** 56, 681.
(68) Mandel, I. D., Cagan, R. S., *J. Oral Therap.* **1964,** 1, 218.
(69) Manly, R. S., *in* "Caries Symposium Zurich," H. Muhlemann, Ed., Hans Huber, Berne, 1961.
(70) Marthaler, T. M., *Brit. Dental J.* **1968,** 124, 510.
(71) Marthaler, T. M., *in* "Caries Symposium Zurich," H. Muhlemann, Ed., Hans Huber, Berne, 1961.
(72) McCormick, J., Koulourides, T., *Intern. Assoc. Dental Res. Abstracts of 43rd General Meeting, 1965,* p. 138.
(73) Mercer, V. H., Gish, C. W., *J. Indian Dental Assoc.* **1968,** 47, 432.
(74) Mercer, V. H., Muhler, J. C., *J. Oral Therap.* **1964,** 1, 141.
(75) Muhler, J. C., *in* "Caries Symposium Zurich," H. Muhlemann, Ed., Hans Huber, Berne, 1961.
(76) Muhler, J. C., *J. Am. College Dentistry* **1968,** 35, 45.
(77) Muhler, J. C., *J. Am. Dental Assoc.* **1962,** 64, 216.
(78) Muhler, J. C., *J. Dentistry Children* **1958,** 25, 306.
(79) Muhler, J. C., *J. Dental Res.* **1958,** 37, 448.
(80) *Ibid.,* **1960,** 39, 955.
(81) Muhler, J. C., *J. Indian Dental Assoc.* **1968,** 47, 428.
(82) Muhler, J. C., Kelly, G. E., Stookey, G. K., Lindo, F. I., Harris, N. O., *J. Am. Dental Assoc.* **1970,** 81, 142.
(83) Muhler, J. C., Radike, A. W., *J. Am. Dental Assoc.* **1957,** 55, 196.
(84) Muhler, J. C., Radike, A. W., Nebergall, W. H., Day, H. G., *J. Am. Dental Assoc.* **1955,** 50, 163.
(85) *Ibid.,* **1955,** 51, 556.
(86) Muhler, J. C., Stookey, G. K., Bixler, D., *J. Dentistry Children* **1965,** 32, 154.
(87) Pameijer, J. H. N., Hunt, E. E., Jr., Brudevold, F., *Arch. Oral Biol.* **1963,** 8, 183.
(88) Peffley, C. E., Muhler, J. C., *J. Dental Res.* **1960,** 39, 871.
(89) Peterson, J. K., Horowitz, H. S., Jordan, W. A., Pugnier, V., *J. Dental Res.* **1969,** 48, 346.
(90) Pickel, F. D., Bilotti, A., *Ala. J. Med. Sci.* **1965,** 2, 286.
(91) Pickel, F. D., Block, A., Bilotti, A. G., Pigman, W., *Ala. J. Med. Sci.* **1965,** 2, 288.
(92) "Progress Report Concerning the Current Status of the Self-Application of the Stannous Fluoride–Zirconium Silicate Preventive Dentistry Paste Program for the Mass Control of Dental Caries," *J. Indian Dental Assoc.* **1969,** 48, 317.
(93) Richardson, A. S., Castaldi, C. R., *J. Can. Dental Assoc.* **1965,** 31, 713.
(94) Rosenkranz, F., Torell, P., *Odontol. Revy* **1961,** 12, 267.
(95) Rusoff, L. L., Konikoff, B. S., Frye, J. B., Johnston, J. E., Frye, W. W., *Am. J. Clin. Nutr.* **1962,** 11, 94.
(96) Scola, F. P., U. S. Naval Submarine Medical Center Memo, Report No. 68–3, 1968.
(97) Scola, F. P., Ostrum, C. A., *J. Am. Dental Assoc.* **1966,** 73, 1306.
(98) Ship, I. I., Mickelsen, O., *J. Dental Res.* **1964,** 43, 1144.
(99) Stralfors, A., *in* "Caries Symposium Zurich," H. Muhlemann, Ed., Hans Huber, Berne, 1961.
(100) Stralfors, A. J., *J. Dental Res.* **1964,** 43, 1137.

(101) Swerdloff, G., Shannon, I. L., USAF School of Aerospace Medicine Report—SAM-TR-67-52, 1967.

(102) Szwejda, L. F., Tossy, C. V., Below, D. M., *J. Public Health Dentistry* **1967**, 27, 192.

(103) Thomas, A. E., Jamison, H. C., *J. Am. Dental Assoc.* **1966**, 73, 844.

(104) Torell, P., *Acta Odontol. Scand.* **1965**, 23, 287.

(105) Torell, P., Ericsson, Y., *Acta Odontol. Scand.* **1965**, 23, 297.

(106) Torell, P., Siberg, A., *Odontol. Revy* **1962**, 13, 62.

(107) Toto, P. D., Rapp, G., O'Malley, J., *J. Dental Res.* **1960**, 39, 750.

(108) Volker, J. F., *J. Am. Dental Assoc.* **1948**, 36, 23.

(109) Volker, J. F., Caldwell, R. C., *in* "Clinical Pedodontics," S. B. Finn, Ed., 3rd ed., Chap. 27, W. B. Saunders, Philadelphia, 1967.

(110) Wallace, D. A., *Dental Progr.* **1962**, 2, 242.

(111) Weisz, W. S., *J. Am. Dental Assoc.* **1960**, 60, 438.

(112) Wellock, W. D., Brudevold, F., *Arch. Oral Biol.* **1963**, 8, 179.

(113) Wellock, W. D., Maitland, A., Brudevold, F., *Arch. Oral Biol.* **1965**, 10, 453.

(114) Zacherl, W. A., McPhail, C. W. B., *J. Can. Dental Assoc.* **1965**, 31, 174.


RECEIVED August 15, 1968.

# INDEX


**A**

Absorption of fluoride .......... 98
Acidulated phosphate fluoride ... 163
Adhesion of food products to tooth enamel .................. 15
Adrenalectomy ............... 84
Age .......................... 4
Agents applied by dental team ... 162
Aglycones of flavanones ........ 71
Aluminum .................... 149
Amine fluoride dentifrice ........ 174
Amino acids ................. 23
  *vs.* tooth solubility .......... 30
Amphotericin B .............. 48
Ancient teeth
  of Indian Knoll ............ 132
  of Pueblo Indians ........... 132
Animals
  caries susceptibility *vs.* diet in .. 9
  mineral composition of teeth in humans and experimental .. 129
Animal studies
  antibiotics ................47–9, 74
  carbohydrates ..........8–10, 19, 24
  casein ..................... 25–7
  fats ......................11, 80
  minerals .............117, 126, 139
  organic compounds .....76, 78, 80, 83
  seed hulls .............56–8, 61, 65
  vitamins .................... 42
Anion exchange resins .......... 79
Antibacterial activity
  *vs.* antioxidant activity ....... 73
  *vs.* caries activity ........... 64
Antibiotics .................. 46
Anticaries activity
  from oat hulls ............... 63
  of seed hulls ................ 61
Antienzyme action ............ 174
Antienzymes ................. 73
Antifungal antibiotics .......... 48
Antihistamines ............... 83
Antimycotic agents ............ 48
Antioxidant polyphenol ......... 71
Antioxidants .................72, 86
  organic .................... 73
Application of chemical agents for the control of dental caries .. 161
L-Arginine .................. 28
Artificial
  mouth ....................13, 14
  plaque .................... 48
Ascorbic acid ................ 39
L-Aspartic acid ............... 29
Aureomycin ................46–8, 50

**B**

Bacitracin .............47, 48, 51, 53
Bacteria associated with dental caries relationships ......... 29
Bacterial polysaccharides ........ 53
Bacteriostatic action of the flavanoid class ............ 72
Barium ..................... 149
Basic process in dental caries .... 8
Beryllium ................... 147
Betadine .................... 86
Beverages, fluoride in .......... 97
Biotin ...................... 38
Black treacle ................ 67
Blood fluoride ................ 99
Bone fluoride ................ 103
  deposition, mechanism of ...... 104
Bones, inorganic composition of .. 129
Boron ...................... 146
Bound fluoride ............... 99
Bread, fluoride in ............. 110
Breast feeding, dmft *vs.* ........ 107
Bromine .................... 149
Brown sugar ................. 67

**C**

Cacao factors ................ 69
L-Cadaverine ................ 28
Cadmium ................... 142
Calcium
  and phosphorus ............. 116
  radioactive ................ 137
  *vs.* dental caries development .. 117
Camellia .................... 94
Candy ...................... 15
Carbohydrates ................ 7
Carbomycin .................. 47
Carbonyl-binding
  agents ..................... 76
  compounds ................. 82
Caries
  activity, antibacterial activity *vs.* 64
  and trace elements, geographic variations in ........... 125
  effect, elements with doubtful .. 147
  experience, variability of ...... 20
  in the southwestern states ..... 126
  -inert elements ............. 149

Caries (*Continued*)
  in experimental animals 55
  -promoting elements 138
  studies, materials and compounds cited in 59
  susceptibility *vs.* diet in animals 9
Cariogenic agents
  cereals 25, 118
  hormones 84
  minerals 138
  refined sugar 10, 14, 16, 19
Cariogenicities of foods 66
Cariostatic agents
  amino acids 25, 28, 29
  antibiotics 46–8, 50, 53
  chocolate 68
  fats 11
  fluoride 105–7, 109, 163, 166
  minerals 119, 120, 143
  organic compounds 71, 75–8, 86
  proteins 26, 27
  seed hulls 58, 59, 61, 65
  sugar 67
  vitamins 37
Cariostatic
  elements that are mildly 142
  nutrient, lysine as a 25
Casein 26
  –sucrose ratio 26
Cedar wood 62
Cephalosporin 47
Cereals 24, 65
Chemical agents for the control of dental caries, application of 161
Chelators 86
Chewing gum 176, 177
Children
  dental caries in 107
  phosphates *vs.* dental caries in 121
Chloramine-T 165
Chloramphenicol 48
Chloromycetin 47
Chlorophyllin 78
Chocolate 67, 69
  milk 68
Citric acid content of human teeth 132
Civilization, dental caries *vs.* 123
Cobalt 147
Cocoa 67, 69
  beans 72
  decalcification-inhibitory activity for 69
  powder 68
Complexing agents 77
Composition of outer and inner enamel of teeth 130
Compounds cited in caries studies, materials and 59
Cones 62
Copper 146
  in teeth 133
Cost of dental services 1
Cottonseed hulls 61

## D

Decalcification
  inhibitors 64–6
  -inhibitory activity
    for cocoa 69
    in wheat bran 66
Declomycin 48
Dental caries 1
  application of chemical agents for the control of 161
  basic process in 8
  development, calcium and phosphorus *vs.* 117
  dietary minerals, food ashes, and experimental 126
  distribution of 2
  in experimental animals 5
  factors influencing 4
  fluoride and 105
  in children 107
    phosphates *vs.* 121
  incidence of 2
  minerals *vs.* 123
  relationships
    bacteria associated with 29
    protein associated with 29
    vitamin 34
  role of phosphorus in 118
  saliva and 8
  *vs.* civilization 123
  *vs.* urinary Se 138
Dental team, agents applied by 162
Dentifrices 73
  fluoride 110
  for dental caries, therapeutic 173
  sodium monofluorophosphate 173
Dentinal caries 5
Deposition of fluoride 103
Dextranases 81
Diamox 84
Dietary
  chemicals 1
  minerals and experimental dental caries 126
  pancreatin 57
Diet
  in animals, caries susceptibility *vs.* 9
  New England 127
  plus fluoride 106
  Texas 127
Dihydrostreptomycin 48
Discoloration of the tooth substance 133
Diseases of the mouth 1
Disinfectant cap splint 165
Disinfectants 82
Distribution
  of dental caries 2
  of fluoride 99
Dithiothreitol 73
Diuretic 84
DMFT 2

Dmft
vs. breast feeding 107
vs. sweets 107
Doubtful caries effect, elements with 147
Dried milk 25

E

Echinomycin 48
Edentulous Tahitians 124
EDTA 77
Electron probe 134
Elements
caries-inert 149
with doubtful caries effect 147
mildly cariostatic 142
Enamel
major inorganic constituents of human 131
maturation 136
minor inorganic constituents of human 131
of teeth, composition of outer and inner 130
white spots in the 4
Enzyme 80
activators in microbial cells, metal ions as 128
Erythromycin 48, 52, 53
Ethylenediaminetetraacetic acid 77
Excretion of fluoride 101
Experimental animals, caries in 5, 55

F

Factors influencing
caries 4, 5
effect of minerals on dental caries 150
Fats 7, 10
Fish
meal 96
protein concentrate 26
Flavanoids 79
bacteriostatic action of the 72
Flavanones 69
aglycones of 71
Flavofungin 48
Fluoridated
milk 109
table salt 109
Fluoridation of the diet 169
Fluoride
absorption of 98
administration, other vehicles for 108
agents, self-application of 167
and dental caries 105
blood 99
bone 103
bound 99
diet plus 106
dentifrices 110
deposition of 103, 104
distribution of 99
excretion of 101
food 106
human serum 99
in beverages 95
in bread 110
ingested vs. that in water and food consumed 97
in human diet 95
in plants, inorganic 94
improves tooth health, mechanism by which 110
lozenges 109
metabolism 98
minerals 93
mouthwashes 110, 175
nonexchangeable 99
in the urine 101
skeletal concentrations of 104
tablets 108
–vitamin combinations 108
water-borne 105
Fluorine 93
Folic acid 38
Food
ashes and experimental dental caries 126
cariogenicities of 66
consumed, fluoride ingested vs. that in 97
fluoride 106
fluoride excreted vs. that ingested in 101
intake, frequency of 85
vs. plaque pH 12
French Polynesia 124
Frequency of food intake 85
Fructose 10
Fungi 53
Fungicide sodium dehydroacetate 73

G

Geographic variations in caries and trace elements 125
L-Glutamic acid 29
Glycine 29
Glycolysis inhibition 75
Gnotobiosis 52
Gold 147
Gram positive bacteria 46
Gramicidin 51
Greek teeth, mineral content of 132
Griseofulvin 48

H

Halogen pool 102
Hereditary factors 20
Hexokinase inhibitor 73
L-Histidine 28
Honey 67
Hormonal factors 83
Hulls
peanut 64
seed 56, 57, 61, 62, 65

Human
diet, fluoride in .............. 95
enamel
major inorganic constituents of 131
minor inorganic constituents of 131
nutritional studies ........... 9
serum fluoride ............. 99
studies
carbohydrates .......10, 11, 16, 17
fluoride .....23, 105, 108, 163, 167
penicillin ................. 50
protein ...................23, 24
selenium ................ 138
vitamins ..................35, 37
Humans and experimental animals, mineral composition of teeth in 129
Hydrogen peroxide ............ 73
Hydroxyapatite ................ 136
Hydroxycinnamic acids ......... 69

I

Incidence of dental caries ....... 2
in the southwestern states .... 126
Indian Knoll, ancient teeth of ... 132
Inhibition of tooth decalcification ..................64, 66
Inner enamel of teeth, composition of ...................... 130
Inorganic
composition of bones and teeth 129
constituents
of human enamel, major .... 131
of human enamel, minor .... 131
fluoride in plants ........... 94
Inositol ..................... 38
*In vitro*
caries production ........... 13
laboratory procedures ........ 10
Iodoacetic acid ............... 47
Iodine ...................... 149
Iron ........................ 150
staining properties of ........ 133

J

Japanese shrimp .............. 96

L

Lability of seed hull factors ..... 63
Lactose ..................... 10
Lathyrogens .................. 82
Lead ....................... 142
in teeth .................... 133
Leucoanthocyanins ............ 69
Lithium ..................... 146
Local agents
antibiotics ............49, 50, 53, 73
carbohydrates .............. 8
coarseness of diet ............27, 67
fluoride ......163, 167, 172, 175, 176
gum ...................... 177
organic compounds ...........75, 78
saliva ....................83, 136
Local effects .................. 4
Lysine ...................... 28
as a cariostatic nutrient ....... 25
Lysozyme ................... 81

M

Magnesium .................. 140
Maillard reactions ............ 69
Major inorganic constituents of human enamel ............ 131
Manganese .................. 147
Materials and compounds cited in caries studies .............. 59
Maternal–fetal transfer of $^{18}F$ ... 100
Maturation .................. 136
Mechanism
by which fluoride improves tooth health ................ 110
of bone fluoride deposition .... 104
Mercury, staining properties of ... 133
Metal ions as enzyme activators in microbial cells ............. 128
DL-Methionine ................ 28
Microbial cells, metal ions as enzyme activators in ......... 128
Microbiological assays .......... 55
Milk ....................... 170
fluoridated ................. 109
Mineral
composition of teeth in humans and experimental animals .. 129
content of Greek teeth ....... 132
Mineralization ................ 136
saliva *vs.* ................... 136
Minerals ...................93, 116
on dental caries, factors influencing effect of ............ 150
*vs.* dental caries ...........123, 137
Minor inorganic constituents of human enamel ............ 131
Mode of action of seed hull factors 63
Molybdenum ................. 142
Mouth
diseases of the .............. 1
rinses, fluoride ............. 110
Mouthwashes ................ 73
Multiple vitamin–fluoride tablets .. 166
Murexide ................... 136

N

Natural
diets ....................... 10
food protein ................ 24
Neomycin ...................47, 53
Neutron activation analysis ...... 133
New England diet ........... 127
New Zealand study ............ 125
Niacin ...................... 36
Nickel ...................... 150
Nicotinic acid ................ 36
Nitriles ..................... 82
Nonexchangeable fluoride ....... 99
Nonfat powder ................ 68

Novobiocin .................... 48
Nutritional studies, human ...... 9
Nystatin .................... 48

**O**

Oat hull
  anticaries activity from ....... 63
  factors .................... 61
  total phosphorus of .......... 65
Oleandomycin ................ 48
Organic
  antioxidants ................ 73
  compounds ................ 55
  matrix .................... 86
  phosphates ................57, 79
  polymers of films ........... 79
L-Ornithine .................. 28
Orythromycin ................ 47
Osborne-Mendel albino rats ...... 75
Outer enamel of teeth, composition
  of .................... 130
Over-the-counter preparations ... 172
Oxalate .................... 78
Oxidation
  of phenolic compounds ....... 86
  –reduction potential of saliva .. 73

**P**

Paladium .................... 150
Pancreatin .................... 80
Panthenol .................... 47
Pantothenic acid .............. 38
Parathyroid glands ........... 116
Peanut hulls ..............61, 62, 64
Pecan hulls .................. 61
Penicillin .........46, 48–50, 52, 53, 73
  dentifrices ................ 51
Peroxidase ..................81, 80
Pharmacological activity ........ 82
Phenolic
  acids .....................63, 70
  compounds, oxidation of ...... 86
Phosphate fluoride, acidulated ... 163
Phosphate *vs.* dental caries in
  children ................ 121
Phosphorus
  calcium and ............... 116
  in dental caries, role of ...... 118
  of oat hulls, total .......... 65
  radioactive ................ 137
  *vs.* dental caries development .. 117
Pilocarpine ................. 83
Pit-and-fissure caries .......... 4
Plants, inorganic fluoride in ...... 94
Plaque pH .................. 11
  foods *vs.* .................. 12
Platinum .................... 142
Polymyxin .................. 47
Polyphenols ............63, 70, 71, 86
  antioxidant ................ 71
Population studies ............ 23
Pre-eruptive nutrition
  animal ..................9, 27, 34
  human ...........40, 107, 117, 166
Prophylaxis pastes ............ 164
Protein ...................... 23
  associated with dental caries
    relationships ........... 29
  in saliva .................. 24
  in sera .................... 24
  natural food ............... 24
  synthetic .................. 26
  *vs.* tooth solubility .......... 30
Pueblo Indians, ancient teeth of .. 132
Pyridoxine .................. 37

**R**

Radioactive
  calcium and phosphorus ...... 137
  isotopes .................. 133
Rats
  cotton ....................56, 57
  Osborne-Mendel albino ....... 75
  Sprague-Dawley ............. 61
Reducing sugar in saliva ......... 15
Remineralizing mouthwash ...... 176
Rice hulls .................... 62
Role of phosphorus in dental caries 118

**S**

Saliva
  and dental caries ............ 8
  *vs.* mineralization ........... 136
  oxidation–reduction potential of 73
  protein in ................. 24
Salivary glands .............. 83
Salt, fluoridated table .......... 109
Sardines .................... 95
Seed hull .................56–8, 65
  activity ..................61, 63
  factors
    lability of ............... 63
    mode of action of .......... 63
Selenium, dental caries *vs.* urinary 138
Self-application of fluoride
  agents ................167, 168
Sera, protein in .............. 24
Serum fluoride, human .......... 99
Sialogogue .................. 83
Silicon ...................... 149
Silicone oil .................. 80
Silver, staining properties of ..... 133
Skeletal
  concentrations of fluoride ..... 104
  fluorosis .................. 94
Smooth surface caries .......... 4
Sodium
  fluoride ..................47, 166
  iodoacetate ................ 75
  monofluorophosphate dentifrice . 173
  -*N*-lauroyl sarcosinate ....... 73
Softening of enamel surfaces .... 14
Sorbitol .................... 10
Southwestern states, incidence of
  caries in the .............. 126

Spark source mass spectrography .. 134
Speramycin .................. 53
Sprague-Dawley rats .......... 61
$^{90}$Sr ...................... 133
Staining ..................... 133
Stannous fluoride ........135, 163, 168
dentifrices *vs.* reduction in dental caries ................170, 171
Steroid hormones ............. 83
Stickiness ................... 25
Straws ....................... 62
Streptococci ................. 46
Streptomycin ..............47, 51, 53
Strontium .................... 145
Subtilin ..................... 47
Sucrose .....................10, 18
–casein ratio ............... 26
Sugar beets .................. 67
Sulfites ....................77, 86
Sweets, dmft *vs.* ............. 107
Synthetic proteins ............ 26
Syrup ........................ 67
Systemic influences ............3, 4, 8

T

Table salt, fluoridated .......... 109
Tablets, fluoride ............... 108
Tahitians, edentulous ........... 124
Tannins ...................68, 69, 78
Teeth
citric acid content of human .. 132
composition of outer and inner enamel of .............. 130
in humans and experimental animals, mineral composition of 129
inorganic composition of ..... 129
of Indian Knoll, ancient ...... 132
of Pueblo Indians, ancient .... 132
trace element distribution in ... 133
Terramycin .................. 47
Tetracycline ................ 53
Tetracyn .................... 48
Tetradecylamine ............. 80
Tetrahydroxybenzoquinone ...... 79
Texas diet .................. 127
Therapeutic dentifrices for dental caries ................... 173
Thiamine .................... 35
Thiocyanate ................. 78
Thiostrepton ...............48, 53
DL-Threonine ................ 28
Thyroid gland ............... 83
Tin ......................... 148
in teeth .................... 133
Titanium .................... 150
Tooth
decalcification, inhibition of ...64, 66
enamel, adhesion of food products to ................ 15
health, mechanism by which fluoride improves ........ 110
substance, discoloration of the .. 133
solubility, protein and amino acids *vs.* ................ 30
Topical fluoride solutions ....... 162
Trace elements
distribution in teeth ......... 133
geographic variations in caries and .................. 125
Tyrothricin ................47, 50, 51

U

Unrefined
foods ...................... 65
sugars ..................... 67
Urea ........................ 75
Urinary selenium, dental caries *vs.* 138
Urine, fluorides in the .......... 101
Usnic acid .................... 48

V

Vanadium .................... 144
Vancomycin .................. 53
Variability of caries experience .. 20
Vehicles for fluoride administration, other ................... 108
Vipeholm dental caries study ....10, 16
Vitamin
A ........................ 34
B .......................35, 37
C ........................ 39
D ........................ 40
deficiency, effects of ..34–7, 39, 40, 42
–dental caries relationship .... 34
E ........................ 41
excess, effects of .......35–7, 39, 40
–fluoride combinations ........ 108
K ........................ 41
mixtures .................. 52
P ........................ 42
supplements, effects of ........ 42

W

Water
-borne fluoride .............. 105
consumed, fluoride ingested *vs.* that in ................97, 101
fluoridation ................. 167
Wheat
bran, decalcification-inhibitory activity in .............. 66
flours ..................... 66
White spots .................. 135
in the enamel ............... 4
Woods ....................... 62

X

Xanthine ..................... 72

Y

Yellow permanent teeth ........ 124

Z

Zinc ......................... 148
bacitracin .................. 47
in teeth .................... 133